# DECENTER
# EVERYTHING

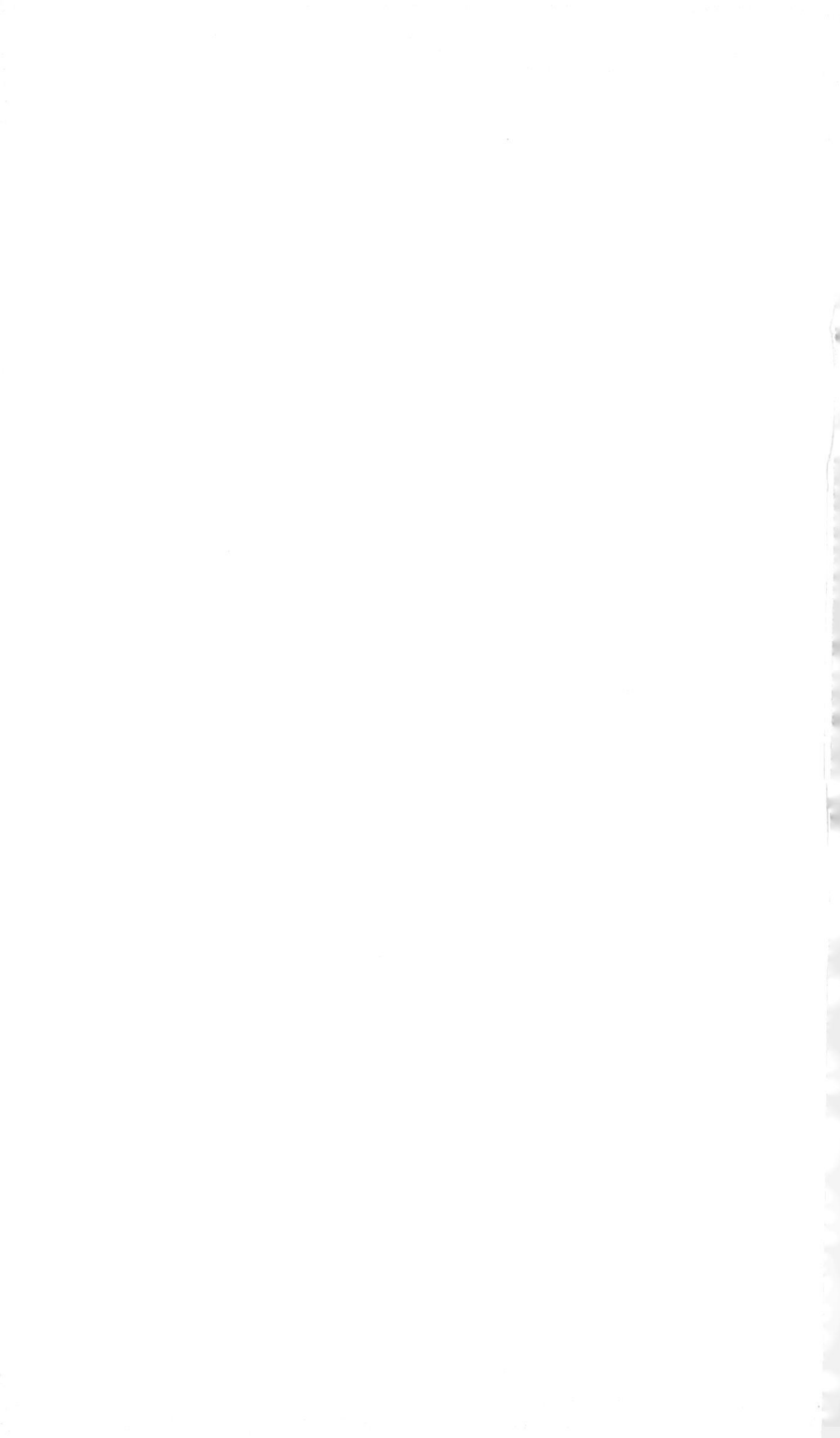

# DECENTER
# EVERYTHING

David Tensen

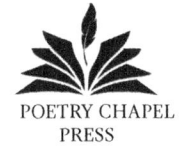

POETRY CHAPEL
PRESS

*Author email: david@davidtensen.com*
*Author website: davidtensen.com*

*Poetry Chapel Press*
*Brisbane, QLD, Australia*

*Cover Design: David Tensen*
*Copy Editing: Rachel Carvosso Mataraki*

*Decenter Everything / David Tensen*

*ISBN 978-0-6456072-4-6*

# DEDICATION

This book is dedicated to Natalie
and our three children.

*You are
my greatest teachers
the most forgiving companions
and source of true joy*

*My deepest thanks to the many beta-readers, draft-readers,
and thoughtful commenters
on the early drafts of this book.*

*Your collective contribution carried this work
through to completion.*

# ENDORSEMENTS

This book not only masterfully explores a vital topic, but is important to me personally. I was affirmed, but more important, deeply challenged. It called me to 'look, listen, and learn,' and offered an invitation to be a grander, more loving presence in the world, especially as I approach the winter of my life.

*Paul Young. Author The Shack. (Over 20 million copies sold)*

Having crossed the threshold of sixty years, my felt need for guided 'eldering' is acute. The disorientation around aging in the face of a shortening future to be expected, and I'm recognizing how the decline in health, energy, work, and potential losses (e.g., of a spouse) lurk in one's mind. I've become convinced that my capacities twenty years from now will depend on how I reorient myself today. But I needed David to suggest 'decentering' as the surprising solution for meaning-making. Decenter Everything! Who knew? I'm all in.

*Bradley Jersak. Principal, St. Stephen's University Author of Out of the Embers: Faith After the Great Deconstruction*

David Tensen is a poet, soul-whisperer, and spiritual provocateur whose words carry the weight of experience and the wonder of transformation. Decenter Everything isn't a book you read - it's a mirror, a mentor, and a map. It invites us to a path that many of us instinctively long for but rarely name: the way of becoming more by centering less.

*Jason Clark. Author of God Is (Not) In Control, and host of Rethinking God with Tacos Podcast. www.afamilystory.org*

Blending personal and spiritual insight, multidisciplinary research, and deep compassion, Decenter Everything is a timely and much-needed guide for the journey toward true maturity. If you've ever longed for a generous elder soul to bless your path, David's words offer deep comfort and practical guidance. I anticipate returning to it again and again.

*Jonathan Puddle. Author of You Are Enough: Learning to Love Yourself the Way God Loves You*

This is a book I will return to again and again - not only for its wisdom and insight, but for the grace and hope it offers. It reminds us that the role of a decentric elder is not just honourable - it is a sacred gift to be shared. Read it. Reflect on it. You may never see your own journey the same way again.

*Dr. Glenn Williams. CEO. LCP GLobal.*
*Author of When Leaders Are Lost*

David is a thoughtful and perceptive soul; well-read, deeply reflective, and endlessly compassionate. Many know him as a gifted poet and writer, but fewer realise the depth of his experience as a counsellor and guide, having spent countless hours walking alongside others, especially leaders, through their own seasons of transformation. Through this book, David guides us toward a life of deeper meaning and purpose, one that is found not in self-centredness, but in embracing our interconnectedness and our calling to support and uplift others.

*Gary Grant - Senior Leader*
*Friends First Community, Melbourne, Australia*

How can the wonder we feel under a clear night sky become a way of life? How can our lives sing with the wild at daybreak? How can we face our last sunset with grace and gratitude knowing we lived well? David's invitation into "decentric wisdom" is desperately needed in an age of acquisition where the promise of greatness has come at the cost of the earth, the expense of the poor, and an alienation from our own soul. I commend David to you as a companion in the work of finding our lives by losing them in the generative service of others.

*Jarrod McKenna. Award Winning Social Change Educator,*
*Activist and Pastor. jarrodmckenna.com*

# TABLE OF CONTENTS

# FOREWORD
By Tara Boothby

I met David Tensen in 2023. At first, I didn't know what reaching out to him would mean for my life. But, connecting with David and asking him for advice has become a journey of knowledge-sharing and a deep blessing as he kindly offers wisdom and support.

> *Realizing we are approaching a learning curve*
> *and seeking support*
> *from a stronger, wiser, other, is leaning into eldering;*
> *eldering is 'leaning in'.*

David is an expert in many ways, and for me I needed help around publishing. David agreed to impart wisdom for my publishing journey, but David did not just pass on information to me, he spent time with me, he corresponded with me, he shared his humor and frustration, his opinions and his humanity. David then met me in my own woes and fears, my excitement and endurance. He was available to me; during our focused project, David was accessible to me; he was responsive to me; he was emotionally engaged with me (in my world as an experiential attachment focused therapist, this is a great big offer of love and relationship).

Eldering is not a pause on the journey, eldering is journeying with another for a time, and then, even if time limits the intimacy of relationship to continue, the legacy, and the energy of the eldering remains - love watches between us while we are apart one from the other.

David has become a friend like this to me: he is my mentor, he is my brother, he is accepting of my neurotic moments, he encourages my strengths, he makes time for me, he teaches me, he is friendly and loving toward me. I am a better person by David's eldering. David embodies the wisdom he encounters and he passes it on.

*Eldering leaves fingerprints on the lives of others.*

Although we have limited ability over what wisdom people take from us, or what information people will retain from the knowledge we impart, I strongly believe that: Interesting people are interested in interesting things.

Being interested in life and gathering interests, then enduring to live with passion for life, interesting people carry life in their body as if it is fire. When they are weary of holding it in, if they are brave, they may find a friend on the trail and bless them by sharing their passion and flame for life. As such, I believe curiosity is a superpower of eldering.

David is always interested and so he is always interesting. He has a breadth and depth of knowledge and interests, and he leans into conversations with others to pique curiosity. My assumption is he enjoys piquing his own curiosity just as much as he enjoys piquing the curiosity of others, and whomever the lucky counterpart, they will be benefited by being in communion with David.

*Eldering is wisdom gathering;*
*Eldering is wisdom sharing;*
*Both.*

It is worth noting, that in our current Western culture, a good deal of individuals strive to live apart from community. Many are choosing to live individualistically.

As a result, we are losing our collective community; we are losing our collective experience more, and self-focused living is prioritized. How much more community will we lose if we do not unpack the practice of eldering and relearn to gift ourselves to others? Eldering holds us accountable to living in community, and so it is strange to wonder how some cultures are losing the practice of thinking together through conversation and interaction.

> *Eldering happens in conversation. Eldering happens in*
> *community with others.*

When we get into the habit of doing things on our own it can be hard to ask for help; Lord knows, I know. When we get in the habit of thinking and taking action independent from others, it can be hard to trust for help; Lord knows I know this as well. Leaning in and relearning to look for wisdom in others takes courage. And then, what is magical about eldering is that it occurs in reciprocal relationships.

> *Eldering blesses us mutually to*
> *Learn,*
> *Relearn,*
> *Discover, and*
> *Rediscover,*
> *In connection,*
> *With another.*

> *Eldering is connection with others*
> *and connection is how we survive.*

What we discover from theories of human science is that we are biologically knit with a deep need for relationship. Relationships are essential for our survival. We have a biological makeup that is literally made up of our nature (our state of being), and our nurture (our need for relationships to help our state of being survive and thrive).

*We are knit to be in relationship and to
help others survive, this is eldering too.*

When we get out of the habit of living in a community of relationships we can begin to live behind veils of self-protection, limiting our dependency on others, and so, dismissing our natural biological instinct to lean on a "wiser, stronger, other." How gravely are we omitting, or ignoring, our deep longing and natural instinct for sacred connection with others?

I have heard it said that when we are in peril, when we have no choice but to reach for help, we do. And in the absence of a safe hand being offered, we will grab hold of any hand. When we live in individualistic disconnection, there are fewer safe hands we may reach for. When we live with limited community we have limited insight into what is safe and what is unsafe, whom is helpful, and whom wills to harm us.

*Eldering is offering a safe hand,*
*Being safe for others,*
*When one can,*
*As one can.*
*To model;*
*To reflect an image*
*Of a safe person*
*Embodied.*

*Eldering imparts the practice of safe community.*

*Good eldering breeds good eldering into others.*

I suggest that eldering can be expressed in a variety of ways. And, I urge that it is good to consider how we have offered and experienced eldering in our own lives. Here are some of my suggestions:

Coming along side of another, being in proximity to another, being in conversation, listening and learning, listening and speaking, gathering wit and wisdom, living your age, speaking from your years, collecting experience, setting time to learn, setting time to teach, being embodied, growing yourself, growing with others, growing others, offering a hug, a shoulder squeeze, a wink, a laugh, a shared cry, journaling, writing books, writing poetry, singing songs, being interested in life, and then, loving your own life so you can hear others with loving ears, see others with loving eyes, and know others with a loving mind.

> *Eldering is loving and valuing yourself so you can love and value another.*
> *Eldering is rooting into another for the budding of new growth.*

David Tensen has been an elder, a mentor, and a safe hand for me. I trust the book you are about to read, because I trust the man who has written it.

I want to be clear: I read David's book *Decentering Everything* as a true manifesto of one who embodies the practice of eldering.

May we discover, all the more, how to not succumb to simply aging.

Instead, may we discover how to flourish into eldering.

Tara Boothby

Tara Boothby is a Registered Psychologist in Alberta and British Columbia in Canada. She has been in practice as a people helper, leader, and trainer for over two decades. Tara is the author of "Love and Love's Energy: How Attachment Science Proves That Love Nurtures Our Biological Nature, Impacts Our Positive View of Ourselves, of Others, and of God, and Teaches Us All How to Love." (2024)

# PREFACE

I do have two requests from my readers. Firstly, I ask that if you have the time and willingness, you might write to me and let me know your thoughts and questions from the book - they matter to me. My email address is david@davidtensen.com. I will make efforts to read and reply.

Secondly, I ask that you consider context when it comes to eldering and the knowledge within this book. Why? Because context pays attention to time and place. Without context, we are prone to fall prey to the loudest and largest voices in the room. Without context, an arsenal of cheap parroted definitive answers are likely to stifle and stunt us when given in response to sacred, important, and costly questions. It is the naive, immature, and uninitiated soul who believes they can confidently and succinctly answer questions like "What does it mean to be a man?" or "What does successful parenting look like?" or "What does a good elder look like?". The wise and mature answer to these kinds of questions is, "It depends on the context." What it means to be a married grandmother of 12 grandchildren in her late 50s eldering in a Kenyan village cannot be fairly compared to what it means to be a single college professor in his late 60s eldering in New York City. Race, colour, gender, culture, age, sexuality, time, profession, material wealth, and so many other factors must be taken into account. With context and nuance in mind, I ask you to forgive me for not providing single and simple definitions of the practice of eldering.

While we are here, at the beginning, speaking of context, I think it's important to let you know a little about me. Knowing the following, you might be able to further forgive me, or call me out, for the unseen biases and shortcomings you are likely to encounter in this book. I am a middle-aged, white, cisgender, heterosexual male. I currently live on Gubbi Gubbi land on the Sunshine Coast, Queensland, Australia. I've been together and married for close to 30 years to the same person, Natalie. My parents are immigrants from the Netherlands. My mum worked as a nurse. My father worked as a mechanic and small business owner. I am the eldest of three kids. I lived with Natalie and our firstborn in Japan between 2006 and 2008. The birth of every child we had, including those that didn't make it to full-term, was traumatic for us; Natalie carries precious scars on her body.

I left school early at 16 to work with my father. Later in my late 30s I entered higher education completing a Bachelor's Degree in organisational leadership. I enjoyed studying so much, I went on to do a Graduate Certificate in research methodology, including an Honours degree in business research. I did well enough to get a scholarship and, at the time of writing this, I am halfway through a PhD program – which in Australia spans around three to four years. I am researching small business education through a social learning lens. Throughout the year I teach in the School of Business and Creative Industries at the University of Sunshine Coast. When I'm not working or studying at the university, I work two days per week as an aged care chaplain, providing spiritual care to the disabled, aged, and dying. Working between places of aspiration and expiration is formational, to say the least.

In a small and unique way, working with the aged and dying has also exposed me to the final stages of life, which some residents describe as the final station, the sunset years, or the winter season. There are severely disabled residents in our care, spanning from their 50s into their hundreds. Today, my daughter, my wife, and I work in the aged care sector. My mum was an aged care nurse for close to 50 years.

I became a Christian at 17, met Natalie at 18, got engaged and married just shy of 20. I always felt a deep spiritual call to serve God in some way, and that inner drive has allowed me to experience and live in a world with an awareness of both the seen and unseen. Several years ago, after suffering with severe compassion fatigue, I started to write poetry. It did very well. I've since written four volumes of poetry and helped others write and publish their work too.

My wife, Natalie, was a stay-at-home mum for many years. Being present for our kids was something we valued, but it was also a choice made for us as she accommodated birthing trauma in her body for many years – up until she had surgery in 2018. She studied the social sciences and has worked as a counsellor, and in mental health.

I am what some might call a generalist, or a multipotentialite. It has taken me some time to get over the embarrassing fact that my working career has encompassed many sectors and many industries, and as a result, I carry many skills.

Other random facts: I collect typewriters. I play pickleball. I've been eating a predominantly plant-based diet since I was 40. I am an ENFP on the Myers-Briggs and a 9 on the Enneagram. I love coffee and fine vegan chocolate. I still struggle to call myself a writer, a poet, an academic, a researcher, or any such title.

I have witnessed healing miracles. Not just by way of physical healings, but profound divine encounters that have melted away, and brought healing to, lifelong trauma. I have had profound deeply personal and transformative spiritual experiences – particularly in therapeutic settings. These experiences make it hard for me to be a materialist. I believe in an unseen realm. I've experienced it. And it has shaped the way I see life. Recently, I've grown fond of Alfred North Whitehead's process and relational philosophy, and accompanying theology.

When my youngest son asked me what this book was about, I knew I had to wrap my answer into quick simple language a teenage brain could understand. My response? "It's about growing older without being a dick." My son and anyone close to me know that I haven't arrived. They know I can be a dick at times. Please don't read this book assuming I am without flaws. I have decades to go and am a work in progress. I simply refuse to get older without working on myself so I can handle more of life's messiness, remain anchored to my true self, and create space for others to be their authentic selves too.

My prayer is that this book finds you when you need it most and that you will take note of all the emotions, provocations, and call-to-actions that emerge in you. This world needs more intentional, authentic, and dedicated elders – not just old people.

Love and blessings,

David Tensen
david@davidtensen.com
www.davidtensen.com

## A note on references and spelling.

There are many authors and texts referenced throughout this book. I have placed a reference list, recommended reading, resources, and more on a dedicated page on my website. It can be accessed here:

www.davidtensen.com/decenter

Much of this book uses British English spelling conventions, however I opted to use the US Spelling for the words center and decenter.

# INTRODUCTION

The elders have left the village, and we hardly noticed their departure. This exodus wasn`t marked by ceremony or collective grief; it unfolded gradually and invisibly, as the perfect century-long storm of wars and progress transformed the landscape of ageing in the West into some kind of endless summer for the soul. The result? We've inherited a cultural wound so deep that many of us approaching our autumn years (50 yrs +) can scarcely recognise it, let alone name it.

Author of Die Wise, Stephen Jenkinson, names this wound, suggesting that we're facing not simply a crisis of elderhood, but its near-complete conquest by a culture of age without ageing, retirement without ripening. The post-war generation, our Baby Boomers, inherited a fractured lineage. Their own elders, shaped by depression and war trauma, often carried a stoic silence that masked deeper psychological developmental arrest (immaturity). These were traumatised men and women who survived by compartmentalising, by pushing forward, by refusing to look back – a psychological strategy that served them in crisis but failed to nurture the soulmaking necessary for true elderhood.

Dr James Hollis reminds us that this developmental crisis stems from our culture's profound misunderstanding of life's second half. We've created a society that promises endless youth, endless consumption, endless distraction – anything to avoid the necessary descent into what Franciscan priest, Richard Rohr, calls life's "second simplicity". Author and researcher Sharon

Blackie suggests this avoidance manifests differently yet has had a devastating impact across genders – while men flee from the confrontation with mortality, women are often denied even the cultural space to age authentically, pressured instead to maintain a perpetual spring in defiance of their rich autumn wisdom, made biologically clear through years of menopausal transition.

This perfect storm has produced what might be history's first elderless generation: the Boomers, caught between their traumatised parents and their own unresolved and unintegrated youth, never witnessing genuine elderhood in action. Instead, they saw retirement – that peculiar modern imaginative invention that transforms the autumn and winter season of life into an extended adolescence, complete with its focus on leisure, consumption, and self-referential pleasures.

The consequences of this developmental vacuum are far-reaching. Author of Nature and the Human Soul, Dr. Bill Plotkin's work reveals how this absence of authentic elderhood has ruptured our relationship with the very planet of which our souls are part of, creating generations of developmentally arrested adults who mistake financial security and environmental dominance for psychological maturity and progress. We have lost the ecological consciousness that traditionally emerged through the ripening process of genuine elderhood, replacing it with what Stephen Jenkinson calls "elderly idealism" a state of perpetual youth-mindedness that resists the gravitational pull toward genuine maturity.

For those of us now crossing the threshold into life's autumn season - meaning, the post-parenting, post-reproduction stage of life (around 50-years-of-age) - this transition is both a wound and an invitation. We stand at a crucial developmental crossroad: we can either perpetuate the pattern of stunted emotional, psychological, social, spiritual and ecological development that has characterised recent generations, or we can choose a more challenging path – one that requires us to rebuild and reimagine elderhood and the very practice of eldering. This is no small task, because like most of those born in the 20th century who had to largely parent themselves, we must now learn to elder without elders.

We cannot, however, simply blame the wars and consequential trauma for our present elderless situation. The crisis runs much deeper than generational dynamics. The post-war economic boom, combined with rapid technological advancement, created a convergence of factors that severed the natural transmission of deep wisdom between generations. The traditional apprenticeship in elderhood that was once transmitted through daily interaction, shared work, and intentional mentoring – was replaced by retirement communities, leisure activities, and the segregation of ages that characterises modern life. This segregation has created what amounts to a developmental dead zone – where the crucial tasks of late-life individuation are replaced by what the renowned psychologist Carl Jung warned against: *the tragic attempt to live life's afternoon by the program of life's morning.*

Yet within this crisis lies opportunity. As we face global challenges that demand large levels of wisdom and mature consciousness, the task of reclaiming and reimagining elderhood becomes not just a personal developmental imperative but a collective ecological necessity. The question facing us isn't simply how to age well individually, but how to pioneer new forms of eldering suitable for a world facing crisis. Can we bridge the chasm between our inherited patterns of stunted soul development and the demands of our current planetary and societal moment?

This manifesto (of sorts) emerges from this felt necessity. It's a call to those approaching or inhabiting life's autumn season to undertake the difficult work of breaking the patterns of arrested development (aka immaturity) that have characterised recent generations. It's an invitation to engage in what I have come to call "decentric eldering" – a concept I unpack slowly throughout this book.

To conclude this introduction and prepare for the following chapters, I want to share a poem. This was one of the first poems I wrote when *poetry found me* in 2018. I wrote it while on a small family break near the border of Queensland and New South Wales. Someone gifted our family a week in their timeshare apartment. It could not have come at a more perfect time. I was suffering from compassion fatigue after years of travelling as a sort of *healer* among a number of Christian churches. This poem, Elders, was the cry of my heart during this season, and a cry I hear among many others approaching midlife.

*The campfire-till-coal talks*
*The long-ride-home talks*
*The coffees-until-closing talks*
*These are the conversations my generation thirst for.*

*Elders, where are you?*

*Why are you not listening?*
*When did you get stuck?*
*Where does it hurt?*
*Who told you that your scars*
*and tears and unveiled fears were worthless?*
*For they are priceless.*

*Elders, where are you?*

*Please, don't reach down for relevance.*
*Don't slow down or stop on life's journey*
*through valleys of darkness and death.*
*We need to know what happens next.*

*Elders, where are you?*

*Has materialism won your heart?*
*Has accumulation bewitched you?*
*Has security stolen your courage?*
*Please, tell us we're wrong.*

*Elders, where are you?*

*Or, are we not looking, or asking, or listening for your*
*wise ways?*
*Have we been blinded by youthful hubris and rugged*
*independence?*
*Have our silent cries been silenced by roaring progress*
*into loftiness?*

*Elders, where are you?*

*Please, make yourselves known.*
*Seek us. Find Us.*
*And we can grow up together.*
*Old together.*
*Wise together.*
*Elders together.*

*'Elders'*
*By David Tensen*
*The Wrestle (2020)*

# Opening questions
# for reflection and discussion.

"The elders have left the village, and we hardly noticed their departure." What evidence do you see of this phenomenon in your own communities or cultures? How has this departure impacted society?

How might you recognise the "cultural wound" described in the book within yourself or in others around you? What forms does this wound take in your life?

How does the description of the "perfect century-long storm" (wars, trauma, economic changes) resonate with your understanding of how elderhood has changed over generations?

In what ways might Baby Boomers have "inherited a fractured lineage" and never witnessed "genuine elderhood in action"? How might this generational experience differ from those before or after them?

What examples of the "hollowing out" of eldering practices have you observed in your communities?

What does the poem "Elders" at the end of the introduction evoke in you? Which lines resonate most strongly with your experiences?

How might you respond to this moment described as both "a wound and an invitation"? What invitation do you see emerging from this crisis of elderhood?

# BEYOND AGE AND OFFICE

You, the reader, may have a history with the word 'elder'. I know for some, this word immediately conjures up an older person; depending on what age you are, an elder may range anywhere from 50 to somewhere in their 80s. If you ask an 8-year-old child what an elder is, they may point out their 58-year-old grandmother as an elder. If you ask a 50-year-old what an elder is, not many of them would likely say they are elders; instead, they are most likely to point towards somebody a few decades older.

Language is, and will always remain, contextual.

The challenge with writing any book is doing your best to keep in mind the cultural context of your desired reader. When I wrote my first poetry collection, I was quite surprised by who read it; age, race, place – they all varied. As such, I have learned that the life of a book is uncontrollable. That said, a writer is encouraged to keep a typical reader in mind, because context is key.

It may not be obvious right now, but this book is largely directed at white Westerners. And by white, I don't just mean the colour of one's body, but more to say the whiteness of our culture, the colonial, institutional, often patriarchal, white dominator culture that I am part of, and you are most likely subject to also. For example, if you are reading this and are part of an Asian, African, or Middle Eastern country and culture, (which equates to over 80% of the world population), you may be scratching your head at some of the things written in this book, because the intergenerational connection and honour for the aged and ageing are natural and normal parts of your culture. You may also not be steeped in materialism, and instead accept that there is more to the world we live in beyond the material realm.

I spent several of my high school years in a very multicultural part of Melbourne, Victoria. Our family had moved to the city suburbs from a very quiet (and white) seaside town, where I had done all my primary school years. Moving to the city gave me culture shock, of sorts. I was one of two 13-year-olds in my Grade 7 class born in Australia. Most of my classmates were born in China, Greece, Italy, India or Lebanon. Sure, my parents were Dutch immigrants and Dutch was my first language, but I was born in Australia – and I looked and sounded like a white Aussie.

Gratefully, I made a lot of Chinese friends in those schooling years. A publisher commissioned me to write a book that was translated into Mandarin several years ago, so I travelled over several times. My exposure to Chinese culture was enough to witness my Chinese friends sometimes being reprimanded with a whack across the back of the head or a slap with a spatula from a parent shouting, "Respect your elder!". To my Chinese friends, an elder was their parents. Many Chinese follow the Confucian cultural practice of "filial piety" (xiào), which requires younger generations to show deference and care towards their elders. This has its pros and cons, particularly in single-child families where the child is born with expectations that they will assume responsibility to care for their aged parents and remain under their consultation throughout their lifetime. In some parts of Asia, filial piety is still enforced by law. In historic times, to not comply could lead to the death penalty for you, and a good beating for your neighbours. Still today, many younger Chinese speak of the immense pressure and burden of this cultural system, stating they felt they were born with a job - to sacrifice all their own dreams and desires in order to give their parents a good life.

Honour for older persons spreads beyond immediate family in many cultures. Several years ago, I travelled to Indonesia. I was working as a leadership training and development manager at an international non-profit organisation and my Indonesian colleague picked me up from my hotel in his car. He had brought his wife and his four-year-old son with him. I had spent a bit of time with this colleague over the years, but it was the first time I was meeting his wife and his child. I hopped in the front seat of the car and was introduced to his wife and his son. And he said to his son, "Say hello to Uncle David." 'Uncle?', I remember thinking: 'How am I this child's uncle? Did I blindly sign a document last month for this guy, agreeing to be an uncle to his kid?' But of course, these terms *uncle* or *auntie* are used in an honorific sense across cultures when addressing older people and adults. Again, this is a collective cultural context. In Australia hearing this same kind of honorific language for older persons is very rare, unless of course you spend time with First Nations Aboriginal and Torres Strait Islander peoples, where respect and honour for older and wiser persons are woven into their language, rites, and rituals.

So, should we adopt these same semantics and systems in Western cultures? Should my teenage sons start referring to every older person as aunt and uncle? Should I, as the eldest son in my family, double my workload, have my parents move in, and prepare to cover all their medical bills? Even if I said yes, I very much doubt it will happen. Partly because we have built economic systems to take care of sick and ageing people. But mainly because our Western culture doesn't include defined titles, roles, responsibilities, and rewards for our 'older persons' or honorific expectations from the broader community. Leaving many of us wondering, 'So, what is an elder?'.

In this book, I'm attempting to push back on a couple of definitions of what an elder is and what eldering looks like in the West. If you handed me a clean slate and allowed me to define what an elder (noun) means, I would define an elder as something different from a title given to somebody older than you, or a title given to any old person, or a title given to somebody who holds a position in a church, tribe, or an institution (religious or otherwise). I would appeal to your soul and ask you to consider the character and actions (verbs) of a particular person. Instead of listing 10 ways to spot an elder (noun)....

I would ask you to consider their emotional and spiritual maturity.

I would ask you to consider how they made you feel when you were with them.

I would ask you to explain how they treat others who are in need, including the poor, the sick, the lonely, those close to death, widows, orphans, animals, and the environment.

I would ask you to describe for me their sense of self-importance, how often they need to remind you of their titles or position in your life.

I would ask you to describe to me the level of forgiveness, grace, and understanding they extend to others.

I would ask you to describe to me what is important to them, and where they spent their time and money.

I would ask you to describe the joy that they carry, the hardships they endure, and how quickly they can return to joy from difficult emotions.

I would ask if there was anything you would be afraid of talking to them about or asking them.

I would ask what they do within their community.

I would ask you to describe their spiritual practices, how they speak about God, or the gods, or spirit, or the divine.

I would ask you to describe to me their friendship circle, what excites them, their capacity to love their enemies, their neighbours and themselves.

By considering these questions of another, or perhaps ourselves, we move away from title, age, or hierarchy. Instead, we move towards consideration of the psychological, social, and spiritual factors and actions in one's life. In health and humanity studies, this is sometimes referred to as 'psycho-socio-spiritual' well-being.

In our time, sadly, people have hollowed out the very practice of eldering, reducing it to either 'ageing gracefully'; that gentle acquiescence to time's passage through acceptance and some description of healthy living. Or they will reduce it to an unhealthy attachment to institutional authority derived from age and office. And by office, I mean the rare titled position of power like a religious authority (e.g. church elder), or (grand-) parent, for example. I suggest that both age and office entirely miss the deeper invitation that true eldering represents.

The practice of eldering is not primarily about age but about capacity. Indigenous cultures often identified potential elders early in life, recognising that the qualities required for authentic elderhood such as broader social and ecological consciousness, psychological maturity, and spiritual depth all required long cultivation. A young person might be recognised for their elder potential decades before their hair turned grey, while an older person might never develop the capacity for true elderhood despite their years. This tradition of young people being identified as elders is still practised across some cultures today. In fact, a lady living in a Kenyan village recently wrote to me explaining her 27-year-old son had moved through several rites of passage rituals and was now a junior elder. She explained, "There are set age groups through which every person passes and the respect, duties, and wisdom of each stage are used to guide the communities in their lives, ceremonies, daily activities, and help with solving any problems or crises. And each 'higher' stage elder mentors those coming after them." Notice how the community bestowed the title of junior elder alongside eldering responsibilities. It is more than a static term.

This is why I speak of "elder-Ing" rather than merely "elders," employing the present participle (-Ing) as we do with "parenting." Like parenting, eldering is a practice that can be developed, refined, and expressed across the lifespan. Neurotheologian and psychologist Dr. Jim Wilder suggests that while parenting centers on the capacity to care for a family, eldering extends to caring for the wider community. This expansion of care beyond immediate family circles marks a key distinction of the eldering practice.

"Decentric eldering" is a term I created in considering a path forward for myself. You won't find the word *decentric* in a dictionary because it is a word I have created – a combination of *de*centered and ec*centric*. I'll explain the word-combination more fully in the chapter titled Decentering God.

Again, if you're looking for a simple list of what decentric eldering looks like, you are going to have to pan for those specks of gold in this book. And I promise you that they do exist. But because I do not live in your body, in your mind, in the context of your life, nor do you live in mine, then I think the kindest and most loving thing that I can do is allow the revelations you need, at this point in time, to reveal themselves as you read and reflect on this provocation.

Therefore, I do not apologise for some of the vagueness within this book. Our collective modern addiction to certainty and being right can afford to be disrupted and decentered. Having said that, there are plenty of absolute statements in the text. There will be plenty to think about and consider. There will be plenty to wrestle with and argue with. I hope to be a companion with you in the reimagining of what maturation and soulmaking look like as we journey together through time.

So, why am I writing this then? Well, I do not think we can afford to simply carry on into our ageing future without reimagining what the practice of intentional and conscious eldering looks like. I am closing in on 50 and my three children are entering their early adult years. My wife Natalie and I have been very intentional with our parenting – in fact, we are part of a generation who have enjoyed amazing resources and research on parenting. Much more than our own parents did. And now I am headed into this next phase of life and I am looking for these same resources, guides, and forerunners. I can tell you now, they are lacking. In fact, I recently searched my university's online library catalogue for books and articles on 'parenting' and the search engine returned over 250,000 results. I searched for "eldering," but fewer than 1,000 articles showed up. Many results included "eldering" because it was a surname! When I extended the search out to 'ageing' and 'elderly', the results improved a little – but I am not interested in research about ageing. Getting old is a default event; decentric eldering only happens through deliberation.

You'll see in the next chapter how we found ourselves in this current eldering abyss; suffice to say, we, in the West, have an opportunity to reimagine what eldering may look like. Now that we are living an average of around 50% longer than our great-grandparents did, our souls should be asking, 'Who am I to spend these post-parenting decades of my life becoming?' We must define ourselves for ourselves or we will be headed into a future with expectations that things will work out the same as they did for our parents and grandparents. I'll be frank, these transgenerational expectations are steeped in ignorance. Economic, ecological, environmental, social, and housing researchers will tell you that we are headed for a very different world than our parents and grandparents lived (and are living in) at their age. Consider alone the population growth from 2.5 billion people in 1950 to an estimated 9.7 billion in 2050.

In her recent manifesto, Imagination (2024), Professor Ruha Benjamin underscores the crucial role that collective and intentional, disruptive imagination must play in creating a future. She draws courage from Black feminist poet Audra Loure who said, "If I didn't define myself for myself, I would be crunched into other people's fantasies for me and eaten alive." I couldn't agree more. If we do not reimagine our future selves, we will be eaten alive – and likely by our own blind consumerism!

Friends, we cannot live in the imaginations of our parents and grandparents when it comes to eldering. We must embrace a deliberate cultivation of expanded consciousness and care for all things. We must embrace eldering practices that move in the opposite direction to the 'self-as-center' consumerist mindset that has paraded as the 'elderly-idealism' of the West. Our path forward requires us to envision a world where true wisdom comes not from placing ourselves at the center, but from settling into the circle and serving the whole.

To summarise, the crisis of elderhood in our time isn't primarily about the absence of ageing and older people. As a chaplain in the aged care sector, I can tell you, we have plenty of older people. The crisis is not a lack of people holding positions of power, hoping (or demanding) we submit to their seniority or titles of 'elder' in church, family, and community contexts. The problem is the scarcity of individuals, at any age, who have undertaken the demanding and intentional call of life-long psycho-socio-spiritual maturity. The disturbing truth is that very few people have been guided, supported, and initiated by a community into the kind of necessary self-forgetting and self-emptying soulmaking that decentric eldering calls for.

It is important for us to know and accept that this eldering practice I speak of demands more than just the passage of time, or the accumulation of experience. It requires the courage to grow beyond our culturally inherited individualism. Beyond our need to matter through control or center-stage positioning, into a more subtle and powerful form of presence which, I believe, the soul of creation is groaning for.

Some readers might be asking, "How on earth did we get here? Why are we elderless? And, David, I'm in my 70s and feel a little inadequate, overlooked, and unimportant; are you blaming us for our current condition?" Great questions. Let's explore them.

# Questions for reflection
# and discussion.

How might you distinguish between simply being an "older person" and practising authentic "eldering" based on your own observations?

How does the meaning of "elder" differ across the cultural contexts you have encountered? What can you learn from these differences?

When you consider qualities like emotional maturity, how someone makes you feel, how they treat others in need, etc., which of these qualities do you find most essential to authentic elderhood?

What capacities have you seen develop in yourself or others that might contribute to authentic eldering?

What might a "self-as-center" person look like in practice, and how do their actions effect our understandings of ageing and authority?

How might authentic eldering move beyond both age and office (formal positions of authority)? What could this look like in practical terms in your community?

How does understanding "elder-ing" as a verb/practice rather than being an "elder" as a noun/status shift your thinking about this life stage?

# THE GREAT INTERRUPTION

The erosion of authentic elderhood didn't happen overnight. Multiple cultural forces converged over generations to create what we now face; that is, a profound interruption in humanity's oldest form of wisdom transmission. To understand this loss, and more importantly, to begin reclaiming what's been lost, we must examine these combating forces with sober eyes.

The story begins, perhaps, with the rise of colonial powers and dominator cultures. Nations like Britain, and later America and Australia, built their wealth and identity on a particular form of dominance; over nature, over Indigenous peoples, over the rhythms of life itself. Author Riane Eisler developed the concept of "dominator cultures" versus "partnership cultures" in her 1987 book *The Chalice and the Blade*. She proposed that human societies tend to organise themselves along a spectrum between these two models, with dominator cultures being characterised by rigid hierarchies, male dominance, and authoritarianism, while partnership cultures emphasise more egalitarian relationships and cooperation. This dominance across the globe carried within it a peculiar arrogance: the belief that newer always meant better, that progress was linear, and that the wisdom of the past was merely superstition to be discarded. In colonial societies, particularly young nations like Australia and America, this manifested as a kind of collective amnesia about the very nature of elder wisdom.

Years after this violent and inhumane colonialist history, we see another devastating blow to wisdom traditions across the West: the wholesale slaughter of a generation in the trenches of World War I, followed by World War II. These wars didn't just kill young men and women they eliminated future elders, creating a multilayered tragedy of absence. Those who should have become the wisdom-keepers of the mid-twentieth century lay in foreign fields or returned home carrying body and soul wounds too deep for words.

The numbers alone tell a haunting story, but the deeper impact was cultural and psychological. In Britain, France, and Australia, entire villages lost their young men. As a result, future fathers and grandfathers would never live to share their lives with others. Women were left to raise children alone; their own grief and survival needs often precluding the deeper work of wisdom or soul cultivation. Those men who did return often carried psychological trauma that made the deep connection to loved ones nearly impossible. How does a father teach his child about life's deeper meanings when he's struggling with what we now recognise as PTSD? How does a grandfather share cultural traditions when he can barely speak of his own experiences? How does a grandmother pass on her ancestral knowledge when she's shouldering both grief and the endless practical demands of single parenthood in an increasingly scattered and colonised society?

This trauma echoed through generations. The children of this war-affected generation, the Baby Boomers, grew up in homes shaped by absence and survival. Their fathers were either dead, physically present but emotionally absent, or struggling with war trauma. Their mothers, forced into unprecedented independence, often had to prioritise practical survival over the subtle art of wisdom transmission. Many women found themselves caught between traditional expectations and a new economic realities. Their own elder development was subordinated to the immediate demands of family survival. The chance of any intergenerational wisdom transmission, traditionally passed through extended family networks of both men and women, was largely lost.

Many of these surviving parents found themselves unable to fulfil the traditional elder roles, their own soulmaking stunted by trauma and re-building demands. The stoic silence that characterised many post-war fathers wasn't wisdom; it was wounding. The constant busyness that marked many war-widowed or war-affected mothers wasn't purposeful activity; it was a coping mechanism. This wasn't just about individual trauma; it was about the systematic disruption of wisdom transmission across genders, leaving both men and women struggling to find models for mature development.

This wholesale disruption of wisdom transmission across genders collided with the post-war economic boom, creating a perfect storm of elder-development interruption. My parents, and those born between 1946-1964, dubbed 'The Baby Boomer' generation, came of age in a world of unprecedented wealth and opportunity, but with deep wounds in their inheritance. Their fathers, when present, often sought refuge in work or addiction rather than face their internalised trauma. Their mothers, whether widowed or married to emotionally absent men, had learned to prioritise practical survival over soulmaking.

In this elderless and traumatised vacuum, consumerism offered a seductive substitute for this stifled soulmaking: *status through acquisition.* Why wrestle with the wounds of the past when you could build the future? Why cultivate the subtle gravity of wisdom when you could purchase the trappings of importance? Why engage in the difficult work of elder development when society offered retirement as endless recreation?

This shift affected men and women differently but profoundly. Men, missing models of mature masculinity from their traumatised or absent fathers, often became trapped in patterns of workaholism and emotional unavailability themselves. Women, inheriting their mothers' pragmatic survival skills but missing deeper models of feminine wisdom transmission, often found themselves caught between traditional expectations and new possibilities for independence. Both genders, wounded by their inheritance, turned to consumption and acquisition as substitutes for authentic development.

The result was a generation that achieved extraordinary material success while, according to many developmental psychologists and gerontologists, remained immature in many ways. Their wealth provided immunity from many of life's traditional wisdom-making challenges, while their unhealed familial wounds made them resistant to the very experiences that might have fostered genuine elder development. For most, retirement was not a time for wisdom cultivation and community contribution, but an extended adolescence funded by substantial superannuation accounts and pensions largely funded by the increased taxes their children and grandchildren pay. Inquire of most economists and they will tell you the Boomer generation's wealth creation and sustained lifestyles have never been seen before, and probably won't be seen again. For example, in 2023, American Baby Boomers owned 52% of their country's net wealth despite comprising only 20% of the population. In the US, according to Federal Reserve records, Boomer wealth grew from $4.5 trillion in 1990 to $76.2 trillion in 2023. Boomers now have nearly double the wealth of Gen-X born 1965-1980 and more than five times the wealth of the Millennials born 1981-1996. In short, the current generation of potential elders across the West have been busy booming and enjoying the post-war material spoils at the expense of their own soul growth. Of course, this is a generalisation with outliers, but outliers exist across all generational means and the data is what it is.

The impact of migration adds another layer to this interruption. Take, for instance, the experience of post-war European migrants to Australia and America. Families left behind their homeland and often their extended family networks - the very structures through which elder wisdom traditionally flowed. These migrations, repeated countless times across continents and generations, created gaps in the transmission of cultural wisdom that money and success couldn't bridge. I experienced this familial distance first-hand, along with the majority of my high school friends, whose parents were also immigrants from Europe and Asia. My parents moved to Australia in their late 20s from the Netherlands to start a family. I only remember meeting my eight uncles, aunties, and cousins once. I had two sets of grandparents; one of them moved to Australia when I was young, but that was it. Gratefully, I found substitutes in teachers, sports coaches, church leaders, and in the open homes of solid local families. However, my experience of finding family substitutes generations older than me was not replicated among many of my Asian, African, and European friends who had relatives abroad, with whom they rarely engaged or missed terribly.

Technology has further complicated this picture, accelerating and amplifying what poet and author Robert Bly named "The Sibling Society" – a culture where horizontal peer relationships have almost entirely replaced vertical wisdom transmission. While digital connectivity offers access to information, it has simultaneously eroded the intimate spaces where elder wisdom traditionally developed and was shared. Social media platforms, with their emphasis on peer validation and 'likes', have intensified this flattening of human development that Bly warned about. It has created spaces where almost everyone, except for a popular few elders, speaks as equals, no matter their development or experience. This digital sibling society, as Bly might observe today, creates a peculiar paradox: while we've never had more access to potential wisdom through 'information', we've never been more resistant to the hierarchical relationships through which wisdom traditionally developed and flowed in a kind of 'formation'. Also, social media's democratic nature, (where everyone's voice carries equal weight regardless of development, experience, or wisdom) has inadvertently created what some might call a "wisdom-hostile" environment. Here, the quick wit of youth and snappy attention-eroding production techniques routinely drown out the measured voice of experience. Here, the sustained attention required for wisdom transmission is fractured by endless scrolling and shallow engagement.

Yet perhaps the most insidious force in the West has been the medicalisation and institutionalisation of ageing itself. Marvin Hoffman, writing for the Chicago Tribune in 2014, suggested that retirement communities, while solving certain logistical challenges of ageing populations, have effectively quarantined elders from the broader community. creating *age ghettos* where the vital interaction between generations (once the very medium of wisdom transmission) has been severed . This segregation serves the efficiency demands of capitalism but interrupts the natural flow of intergenerational wisdom. In my own work as an aged care chaplain, I see this social divide up close. I am fortunate that the organisation I work with does their best to create intergenerational connection between those in their care and the wider, younger public. But where I work is the exception, and not the rule in residential aged care centres, in Australia. And the kids who visit from the school next to the village, although kind and polite, are no substitute for familial ties to their own grandchildren.

Please hear me out; our dilemma is by no means a complete absence of elders – they exist, often quietly bringing wisdom into their families and communities. But the systems we've created obscure them. Colonialism marginalised traditional knowledge holders. War decimated many wisdom-keepers. Unfettered wealth elevated retirement over elderhood. Immigration disrupted cultural transmission lines. And now our obsession with digital visibility and youth culture pushes authentic elders further into the shadows – not because they're gone, but because our society systematically overlooks the few that exist.

Finally, it's important to note that this is not simply a personal interruption , it's planetary.  As we face ecological, environmental, and social challenges, the absence of genuine elderhood becomes increasingly critical. The wisdom-keepers and presence of elders that traditionally guided communities through times of change have been replaced by what amounts to a massive cultural blind spot, where those who should be developing and sharing wisdom are instead caught in patterns of consumption, self-centeredness, and distraction. Understanding these interrupting forces isn't about assigning blame but about gaining clarity. This is simply a 'where we are on the timeline right now'. Only by seeing clearly how natural elder development and expression have been disrupted can we begin the work of reclaiming and reimagining eldering for our time. The questions now become: *How do we begin this reclamation in the context of our current reality?  How do we nurture authentic eldering in a culture that seems designed to hinder and prevent it?*

I suggest the path forward isn't found in romanticising some mythical and tribal past. It's not practical to think everyone can go on guided fasts or desert quests for initiation. While these experiences can help many, we must consider how to apply them to billions of people. Instead, I think we need to face the raw reality of our present moment, deeply aware of both our personal and collective stories while heeding the call to maturity. I believe, life itself, has the built-in capacity to initiate us all through stages of necessary maturity, all the way onto the narrow and transformative path of decentric eldering – a path which illuminates based upon our willingness to move aside the things that demand our hearts and skew our perspective on what it means to inhabit the time and age we live in.

# Questions for reflection
# and discussion.

Among the multiple forces that have contributed to the erosion of authentic elderhood, which resonate most strongly with your observations or experiences?

How did the World Wars impact the intergenerational transmission of wisdom? Do you see evidence of this impact in your own family history?

How might consumerism have offered "a seductive substitute for stifled soulmaking: status through acquisition"? Where have you witnessed this substitution in yourself or others?

How does separating ages in today's society, like in retirement communities and age-specific activities, impact the transmission of wisdom between generations?

What examples of the "Sibling Society" (where horizontal peer relationships replace vertical wisdom transmission) do you observe in contemporary culture?

What might it mean to live in a culture of "age without ageing"? How do you see this manifest around you?

How might authentic elderhood address our current ecological challenges? What connections exist between elder wisdom and ecological health?

# FALSE NORTH

If you are reading this, it may be a safe bet that you're not a surface-level, happy-go-lucky, life-worked-for-me, here-for-a-good-time, shit-I'm-awesome, sort of person. You're possibly nodding at what I have penned so far and slightly grieving for the way things are. Like me, you might be somewhere well into, or past, the parenting stage and are wondering what is next because you don't like what you are witnessing ahead and around you. If you are at midlife you may also be wondering why people decades ahead of you seem more like peers and competitors. You might be puzzled as to why simply 'getting old' has become a substitute for being 'an elder', at least in the soulful sense. Something in you is telling you things are not as they should be with the soul of the world. I pray you do not lose this discernment and discomfort. And I pray you gaze across the vista of your own life and inner-wisdom instead of spending your precious energy chasing forms of false elderhood. The cosmos cannot afford this.

When genuine eldering is interrupted, we not only experience an absence of elders, we witness the emergence of various substitutes for authentic elderhood: pseudo-elders. In many cases, these pseudo-elders appear as successful, powerful, and esteemed individuals - and they may be those things. The problem is, all those adjectives denote a subjective outer reality - not an inner state of being. And I argue that decentric eldering is primarily an inside job. We may, as we age, be described as wise according to financial or familial success, power, and esteem. And none of these accolades or achievements are necessarily moral shortcomings or anti-eldering. However, these gains tend to make it harder to dig into the depth of our being that decentric eldering requires. One only needs to read the work of the mystics, poets, and religious figures like Jesus Christ, or the Buddha, to see that the aforementioned trappings (success, power, and esteem) are just that; trappings.

Consider the retired business owner. He struggles to relinquish control of the family business. He views his adult sons, who are educated men in their 40s, as incompetent teens. He believes that his ways, forged in a different economic era, remain the only path forwards. Or the former school teacher who insists her grandchildren should learn, look, and behave a certain way, transforming what could be centered and peaceful demonstrations of loving parental support into an instrument of control every time she visits her daughter and grandchildren. These aren't just personal foibles; they represent a profound constriction of what Dr. Bernard Loomer calls "soul size" – the capacity to hold complexity and difference without feeling threatened.

Loomer defines soul size as "the volume of life you can take into your being and still maintain your integrity and individuality, the intensity and variety of outlook you can entertain in the unity of your being without feeling defensive or insecure." By this measure, many of our substitutes for authentic elderhood actually represent a shrinking rather than an expansion of the soul. They maintain rigid boundaries and fixed viewpoints rather than developing what Loomer calls "the strength of your spirit to encourage others to become freer in the development of their diversity and uniqueness."

After reading Loomer's essay and commentary by Patricia Adams Farmer, I wrote this poem:

*Our souls are a river in flow*
*whose banks and bed are built*
*by every interaction.*
*Whose ways and waters change*
*with every passing breath.*

*I want to be a wide river.*
*Not a narrow brook you simply step over and forget.*
*But wide enough to be considered before crossing.*

*I want to be a slow river.*
*Not an ocean so wild the innocent dare not enter.*
*But slow enough that even the lame feel safe to wade in.*

*I want to be a deep river.*
*Full of life and nourishment.*
*Moving through nations with many streams.*
*Unable to be dammed by dogma or doubt.*

*One day...*
*One fine and inevitable day*
*we will find ourselves emptied out.*
*Emptied out into the Great Ocean of Things*
*adding to it our own minuscule moment.*

*But until that moment.*
*Until the moment my soul ceases*
*to be held as this body,*
*the kind of soul I want to be*
*-I really want to be -*
*is a fat soul.*
*A big fat and generous soul.*

*'Fat Soul'*
*David Tensen (2023)*

Perhaps the most pervasive false adaptation and rigid boundary to cultivating a fat soul and decentric eldering is what we might call "center-stage syndrome" – the persistent need to remain the hero of every story long after the hero's journey should have given way to a more subtle form of enduring presence.

What do I mean by hero's journey? I'll give context to this concept because I will refer to heroic archetypes throughout the book: In the 1940's, professor of mythology, literature, and religion, Joseph Campbell noticed a pattern in many myths and stories, he wrote about this framework which he called The Hero's Journey in his book The Hero with a Thousand Faces (1949). The Hero's Journey is a universal story pattern where a hero (or heroine) leaves their ordinary world to venture into an unknown realm filled with challenges, supernatural aid, and trials, ultimately obtaining a great boon, treasure, prize or revelation through their triumph over a supreme ordeal. After their victory, the hero returns to their original world/home/village transformed by their experiences, bringing back wisdom, skills, loot, or power to their community. However, this return journey often comes with its own challenges of reintegration and sharing their newfound knowledge and transformed selfhood. There are plenty of websites, videos, and books available that unpack The Hero's Journey, suffice to say that Campbell influenced many story-tellers of his time including George Lucas, who adopted the framework for his Star Wars movies. For Christian readers, if you want to see the Hero's Journey played out in the Gospels, Dr. Alexander Shaia has done a wonderful job in his Quadratos books and material suggesting the four Gospels mirror the Hero's Journey pattern. Fascinating stuff.

It may also be worth mentioning that Campbell was influenced by Dr. Carl Jung's work on the collective unconscious. Jung proposed that archetypes are universal, archaic patterns, and images that derive from the collective unconscious and appear in all cultures' myths and stories. Campbell essentially mapped these Jungian archetypes onto the stages and characters of the Hero's Journey. For example, to use the Star Wars storyline, the hero (Luke Skywalker) represents Jung's "Self" archetype – the evolving consciousness seeking wholeness. In Campbell's view, we are all heroes on a journey and this is why great stories are so appealing. We see ourselves in Luke Skywalker, Cinderella, Harry Potter, Bilbo Baggins, Katniss Everdeen, Black Widow, Spiderman, to name a few. Again, there are volumes written on archetypes including some great recent works like Dr. Sharon Blackie's Hagitude (2022) and Gillette and Moore's classic, King, Warrior, Magician, Lover (1990).

However, a growing criticism of the Hero's Journey pattern is that it can oversimplify and force Western ideas onto the rich variety of human storytelling, potentially sidelining cultural stories that don't fit its mould. Many Aboriginal and non-Western stories, for instance, focus on *group* rather than *individual* growth, or move in circles rather than straight lines. Our Western individualistic view perpetuates a bigger problem in today's society: our habit of staying stuck in the hero phase of life rather than growing into elder wisdom. Campbell's ideas help shed light on the importance of life changes and overcoming challenges. However, their popularity may have accidentally strengthened our culture's obsession with personal achievement and heroism. This shift can make it tougher for people to embrace non-hero or post-hero archetypes and transition into their roles as true elders.

The real skill of becoming wise, like Galadriel and Gandalf in Tolkien's Lord of the Rings stories, means moving beyond being the hero to embrace a quieter kind of strength: one based not on personal victories, but on helping others grow, making space for community wisdom, and keeping old meaningful knowledge alive. Galadriel, in particular, shows us how true wisdom includes knowing when to let go of power, as she demonstrates in refusing the One Ring and accepting the end of her time in Middle-earth. This shift of acceptance that our Hero's Journey is ending invites us to cease trying to be the star of every story and instead become what Campbell might call a "bridge between worlds" - someone who has largely completed their own Hero's Journey and now helps others find their way.

I see the inability to let go of the heroic narrative rampant in generations and demographics where material success, titles, and institutional authority often serve as substitutes for genuine soulmaking and authentic elder development. In a desperate attempt to solve (and capitalise on) this eldering void, the personal development industry has been busy offering what amounts to pseudo-wisdom products like boutique overseas tours, weekend warrior workshops, forest retreats, plant medicine experiences, religious conferences, and exclusive spiritual gatherings that promise accelerated enlightenment for the privileged few who can afford the price of admission. While these experiences might offer valuable insights, they often perpetuate the very centricity that authentic elder development must transcend; that being, when elderhood becomes a commodity primarily available to educated, wealthy, and predominantly white-culture individuals, with able-bodies and leisure time, I think we've created another tear in the already fragile fabric of our global community.

Again, it would seem that these false adaptations often share a common feature: they keep the individual firmly at the center of their own universe. I am arguing that healthy development moves in the opposite direction, toward decentric eldering. This isn't about self-rejection or total denial of ego, but rather about expanding the circle of what we hold as precious and meaningful. No thing! not our status, our wealth, our knowledge, or even our spiritual insights belong at the center of our being and identity. Instead, the invitation into authentic eldering is to foster an ever-widening circle of inclusion, care, and consciousness. If you are in life's second half, please understand that we are invited to take on a post-hero position and allow a different archetype to emerge, like we see in the examples of Galadriel, Gandalf, and other mythic characters.

Recently, I took stock of people in my own life who embodied the many post-hero archetypes well. Here is a simple list you might use as a guide when considering those around you, or perhaps the kind of archetype you'd like to develop. The examples that follow are popular story characters of our time.

**Elder Sage:** One who holds wisdom and guides others. Example: Master Yoda – transcended his warrior phase to become a teacher.

**Keeper of Stories:** Guardian of tradition and memory.
Example: The Grandmother in Moana – passes down
cultural knowledge and initiates the Hero's Journey.

**Threshold Guardian:** Protector of sacred spaces and
transitions.
Example: The Oracle (The Matrix) – guides from a
place of seeing multiple possibilities.

**Sacred Fool:** Holder of unconventional wisdom.
Example: Doctor Who – particularly Tom Baker's
portrayal, using apparent eccentricity to mask wisdom.

**Wounded Healer:** One who helps others through their
own scars.
Example: Dr House (TV Show) – helps others while
wrestling with his own pain.

These examples and people moved beyond personal
glory to serve others. They hold paradox and complexity
rather than seeking clear victories. They work through
influence and wisdom rather than direct action. And they
often act as bridges between different worlds or ways of
being.

Perhaps you see yourself in one or more of those
archetypes? Does anyone in your life come to mind? Any
parents, relatives, teachers, sports coaches, neighbours,
scout leaders, pastors, or workplace leaders? If you can
say yes to a few of these, you are blessed – not only to
have them in your life, but to experience what it is like
to be in the presence of those who have moved beyond
*center-stage syndrome.*

The rise of pseudo-eldering is becoming apparent in therapy and counselling rooms. Fifty-somethings arrive with the same existential questions that plague eighteen-year-old school leavers: "What should I do with my life?" Now, if the person were in some kind of induced coma or just lost every dear soul to them to a terrifying Book of Job style disaster, these sorts of questions are very much warranted. But aside from these rare events, we have to wonder what this person has done for three decades of their life – or, to be more direct, what they have done with their soul for three decades. To repeat, psycho-socio-spiritual developmental arrest seems to be so common that we should not be surprised when the masses mistake eldering as an eternal heroic life-building saga centered on a single (monomythic) character: 'me', 'my big goals', 'my wonderful purpose', 'my endless success', 'my numerous holidays', 'my important place in the family`, 'my sacrifice', 'my winning team', 'my expansive plans', 'my troubled existence', 'my faith', 'my great knowledge', 'my victimhood', etc.

Rather than attempting to maintain centricity through control, knowledge, or spiritual achievement, the person growing in a decentered kind of elderhood develops the capacity to hold more. More perspectives, more uncertainty, more ways of knowing and being. This isn't about becoming self-less but about becoming less self-centric. I suggest that decentric eldering is marked by the practice of continually crafting an inner life that Loomer describes as marked by "the power to sustain more complex and enriching tensions."

Now, the accessibility of elder development emerges as a fair concern here. If what we are calling 'true elderhood' can only be achieved through expensive retreats, privileged leisure time, or specific life experiences like parenting, we've created yet another form of spiritual materialism, and perhaps an elite form. Instead, authentic elder development must be available in every context; in poverty and wealth, in illness and health, in families and in solitude. It must be inhabitable: everywhere and always.

To be clear, I would argue that none of these false adaptations to eldering I've described are character flaws to be condemned. Instead, they are stunted aspects of psycho-socio-spiritual growth (developmental arrest) to be understood. In other words, pseudo-eldering points towards both our deep hunger for significance and belonging, plus our profound confusion about how to move forward considering the elderless landscape we've walked into. To begin with, it may be fair to say that if we can recognise these adaptive patterns in ourselves and others, we can move forward by discerning the difference between authentic elder development and its many substitutes. However, there is a catch to all this which certainly lowers its appeal, particularly among the very rich and very religious who tend to buy or bypass their way out of the necessary discomfort truth delivers daily. That is, moving forward beyond pseudo-eldering is no longer an exercise of piety, gain, or acquisition.

Moving forward is not about acquiring more knowledge, more status, more spiritual experiences, etc. Instead, it is about the development of inner-capacity in order to serve the world by divesting all, while remaining authentically *who we are.* To borrow from Loomer again, we gain this eldering capacity throughout life by developing "the magnanimity (generosity) of concern to provide conditions that enable others to increase in stature." Put in simple terms, we must actively find ways to see others grow. In decentric eldering terms, we settle into the circle's edge and make room for others to expand also.

Finally, I think it's important to add that a decentric elder is not necessarily an ascended and leveraged 'expert' person of sorts. (I discuss this in the chapter on Decentering Knowledge). We are also not meant to age into a legacy-bent stepping stone for others, nor a kind of bottomless well of riches for future generations. As Bayo Akomolafe writes so poetically, "The expert... is the elder captured and put to good use. The expert is the elder rendered purposeful, subservient to an already determinate end...the elder (on the other hand) is not useful; the elder is the cautionary delimitation of usefulness." You may need to read that a few times.

This paradox of generous divestment and non-usefulness may take a while to sink in. For me, this is taking a while to metabolise and it seems to be a state of becoming that is gifted through the practice of grieving, humiliation, uncomfortable solitude, and by examining my inner narratives of heroism, victimhood, innocence and villainization – to name a few. Trust me, my ageing ego wants to be appreciated, legitimised, adored, known, remembered, self-sufficient, good, seen and esteemed. One may argue these virtues are not just valid but important contributors to a healthy sense of wholeness, and this is true. When we are younger, moving through the spring and summer seasons of life we need those good and desirable things! However, when (and if) we reach the autumn season of life, which today might be marked at around 50 years of age, we are called to transmorph the posture of our soul. To quote poet Robert Bly:

*It is not our job to remain whole.*
*We came to lose our leaves*
*Like the trees, and be born again,*
*Drawing up from the great roots.*

In my chaplaincy rounds to aged care residents who are mostly in the final months of their winter season, I have become an eye-witness to precious souls of various kinds. Some have great settled roots that you can feel in their presence. Others, however, seem still desperate to stay above the canopy of importance throughout life at the great expense of the others. People who practised forms of authentic eldering often experience the glorious psycho-spiritual phenomena that researcher Lars Tornstam calls gerotranscendence. This means they shift from a purely practical, logical view of life to seeing themselves as part of something larger and more spiritual. As a result, they often feel more satisfied with life. Tornstam uses the words 'cosmic' and 'transcendent' to describe this experience. Some researchers in this field suggest only 20% of people in the West, including those with cognitive impairment such as dementia, experience this state of gerotranscendence in their final years. And what of the 80%? Well, for me and many who work in end-of-life care, we witness the rather sad event of a soul unable to move from center-stage. They spend their last days (sometimes years) sharing exacerbated stories, accolades, gossip, disappointments, and petty complaints like teenagers at school lunch break. I do not know for sure, but research suggests that in other cultures and times, gerotranscendence and the deep embodied and spiritual satisfaction of a life lived well were experienced by a larger percentage of the population.

In conclusion, I would suggest that today, in the West, we are witnessing (and experiencing) the effects of pseudo-eldering and the erosive impact it has had on families, the environment, the economy, and the inner maturity of many. And this trajectory, precious reader, is not sustainable.

In the following chapters, I suggest several things we can each decenter – or keep decentered. Meaning, if we can keep these things on the edge of our soul's inner circle, and not in the middle, we will have a greater chance of becoming what we might imagine. I am going to start with perhaps the most provocative one, Decentering God. Before you close the book and email me for blasphemy, please make your way to the next chapter. It will not only clarify where the term 'decentric' emerged from, but might just be the agitation you need – especially if you identify as a Christian and, like I do, feel the inner pull of the Spirit into generous ways of being and becoming.

# Questions for reflection and discussion

What substitutes for authentic elderhood have you observed in your community or culture?

How might "center-stage syndrome" manifest in older adults you know, or perhaps in yourself? What makes this pattern so difficult to recognise in ourselves?

If "soul size" refers to "the volume of life you can take into your being and still maintain your integrity and individuality," how does this concept help you understand the difference between authentic elders and pseudo-elders?

When have you experienced the distinction between wisdom and knowledge in your life - perhaps receiving wisdom rather than mere information?

What evidence do you see of psycho-socio-spiritual arrested development in your society? How might this manifest across different age groups?

Among the post-hero archetypes (Elder Sage, Keeper of Stories, Threshold Guardian, Sacred Fool, Wounded Healer), which resonates most with you and why?

How might our culture's emphasis on youth and heroic narratives make it difficult to embrace authentic elderhood?

# DECENTER GOD

Much of the feedback that I received when I offered the first drafted chapters of this book to the public was that the picture I painted around the desolation of elders was something that rang true for many. In the midst of those reviewers were a large number of Christians. To be clear, by no means do I think that the 50 people who reviewed and replied to the draft, of whom most were Christians, are a fair sample of the population. However, over one quarter of the world's population do identify as Christians, so I feel compelled to spend some time unpacking a view that I think is important to the practice of decentric eldering – that is; decentering God.

If I am to speak of God in meaningfully Christian ways, I need to take seriously the teaching that the Mystery of God is revealed as the Holy Trinity. Like my Muslim and Jewish friends and neighbours, we too believe God is One. In the life of Jesus, however, I am invited into the experience of the Oneness as "Father, Son and Holy Spirit". Orthodox theologian Kallistos Ware states,

*"There is in God genuine diversity as well as true unity. The Christian God is not just a unit but a union, not just unity but community… God is triunity: three equal… each dwelling in the other two by virtue of an unceasing movement of mutual love."*

I know that most professing Christians, regardless of denomination, hold to the theological view of God as Trinity. A profession of belief in the Trinity exists in many church creeds and doctrinal statements. I would like to say an agreement in the existence of the Trinity is all I need to preface and qualify what I am proposing in this chapter; however, I cannot assume just because we both may hold to a Trinitarian perspective of God that we all see *union with God* in the same way – because there is a chance that we do not. So please bear with me for a few pages as I explain my position so that you can read the rest of this chapter with context for decentering God. If theology or religious nuance is not your thing, feel free to skip this chapter because there is plenty more in this book. In fact, I often wonder if a non-religious view of God simply being *love and a higher power which we return to upon death* is not a decentered gift greater than the tangled box of theological twine most Christians are handed.

Humanity's union with God can be viewed through many theological and doctrinal lenses, but I will give you three perspectives that are common across the global church. There is a good chance that you will feel at home in one of these views. I will include some authors and thinkers, along with scriptures that support the view. Please note that this overview is not exhaustive, nor are the authors mentioned bound to the views I have listed them in; they are just listed indicatively.

**1. Covenantal and Forensic Union** is commonly found in the Reformed & Evangelical Traditions. This view emphasises Union with Christ as a legal, contractual, relational, and covenantal reality. The believer is joined to Christ in a manner likened to a marriage contract, where the two remain distinct but are bound together by divine decree. Scriptures that support this view include Romans 5:12-21 (federal headship) and Ephesians 5:22-33 (marriage imagery). This perspective sees one's union with God as primarily representational (Christ acts on behalf of the believer), judicial (Christ's righteousness is imputed), and covenantal (secured by divine promise rather than mystical participation). Key thinkers include authors like John Calvin, Louis Berkhof and Jonathan Edwards.

**2. Mystical and Ontological Union** is commonly found in the Eastern Orthodox and Catholic Traditions. This view sees Union with Christ as a profound mystical participation, where the believer is drawn into the divine life itself. The language of interpenetration (perichoresis) suggests a sharing in the divine energies (Orthodox) or the process of deification (theosis). Scriptures that support this view include 2 Peter 1:4 ("partakers of the divine nature"), John 15:1-5 (vine and branches), and much of John 17 (pre-cross confession of union v22-23). This union is not just forensic but transformational. In this view of union, believers are gradually divinised, sharing in God's very life without becoming God in essence. Key thinkers include Athanasius of Alexandria, Gregory Palamas, Thomas Aquinas, John of the Cross.

**3. Existential and Relational Union** is found in more Modern Theological Perspectives. Key Thinkers include Karl Barth, Jürgen Moltmann, T.F. Torrance. Barth and Moltmann saw Union with Christ not merely as forensic or mystical but as existential participation in Christ's history and suffering. This view emphasises that Christ's life becomes the believer's reality. Scriptures that support this view include Galatians 2:20 ("It is no longer I who live, but Christ who lives in me"). Here, the union is deeply relational and personal rather than contractual or metaphysical. It focuses on the believer's lived experience of Christ's faithfulness rather than an external imputation or mystical absorption.

As mentioned, there are many other views and variations of these three models of union, but it is worth noting that most Evangelical churches across the West, default to the first view of union in this list: Covenantal and Forensic (legal). This often includes reformed, revivalist, and individualistic beliefs on salvation. If this is your experience and background, what I am suggesting in this chapter may seem a little confusing or heretical because my approach here comes from Christian traditions many centuries older than the others; that being the Mystical and Ontological Union perspective (no.2), which also may be integrated into the third view in the list.

To repeat, this view of mystical union and non-separation between Christ and creation is not new. Please don't bother writing to me accusing me of a new-age view of God. For context, Athanasius of Alexandria and early church theologians like him were born in the 4th century. Calvin and others like him developed their views on 'separation from God until made legally right' more than a millennium later, in the 16th century. It is possible that the legal and contractual view of union with Christ hasn't helped with the maturity of elders, as I am advocating. Why? Because dualistic separation introduces the possibility for my very being to be separated from Christ. Whether Calvin and others intended it, the legal and contractual view of union has morphed salvation into an individualist heroic pathway, and this places immense power on one's ability to overrule God's eternal redemptive work through our mental ascent, measured belief, and the maintenance of a promise to love and obey.

For Bible lovers, this mystical union and view of being can be found throughout the scriptures. Here are some key verses:

2 Peter 1:4: participating in divine nature

John 15:1-5: the vine and branches

John 17:20-23: mutual indwelling

Romans 8:9-11 & 31-39: the Spirit's indwelling and no separation from Christ's love

1 Corinthians 6:17: one spirit with the Lord

Colossians 3:3-4: life hidden with Christ

2 Corinthians 3:18: transformation into Christ's image

1 John 3:2: becoming like Christ

Romans 6:3-5: baptism into Christ's death and life

Ephesians 2:5-6: raised and seated with Christ

Colossians 1:27: Christ in you

Philippians 1:21: "to live is Christ"

2 Corinthians 5:19: reconciliation of the world

You can visit the reference link at the end of the book for recommended reading on all this.

Now, for context, I started my personal faith journey in the first camp. I saw union with God largely as a legal and positional matter. I wanted to be 'saved' and wanted to know what necessary steps could be taken to ensure that I was in right standing with God. My starting position was that of fear and separation. Throughout my life, I believed that I had to keep up my end of the deal, adhering to the rules and laws handed down from religious leaders. Much like a little boy wanting to be good and not risk estrangement from authority figures, I played the family game and it worked for a good 15-20 years. However, it was disrupted by three main things. First, I started encountering Christ in a very spiritual and personal way – and He was far kinder, loving, and understanding than I had been told. Second, I began working with abuse and trauma survivors in a therapeutic capacity. Third, I started reading through the works and commentaries of early Church Fathers.

Without really knowing it, I had moved to an ontological perspective (a view of nature itself) that started and ended in Union with Christ (regardless of what my conscience told me). This was not just good news for me, but amazing news for the world around me. Why? Because it removed the belief that separation from God was possible or conditional. Because salvation was something for me to work out, not work in (Phil 2:12). Because I was able to see Christ in all creation

(Acts 17:28). Because I don't see the work of Christ as inadequate, and I therefore don't view other people as a save-you-from-hell project (2 Corin 5:19). I don't see God the Father as a blood-hungry angry dad with an anger problem (1 John 4:7-12). And if you ask my close family and friends, they will tell you I have become more loving and genuine. But to get here, I needed to let go of the many expectations and images I had of God. Perhaps the best way to explain this is with a poem I wrote around Easter 2019, several years ago. It is called Kind of Way.

*I know that you know.*
*So I should probably confess it.*
*Not because it's a bad thing.*
*But because it's normal*
*and necessary to admit*
*you've disappointed me*
*and continue to.*
*Although I don't mind as much*
*now.*

*Still, there were many times*
*I prayed.*
*Followed the rules.*
*Gave my two mites.*
*Did all the things I was told would work*
*and others certified*
*with charismatic conviction*
*to do more*
*give more*
*faith more*
*sacrifice more*
*lots more.*

*But still, nothing.*
*No breakthrough*
*like I believed*
*like I prayed for.*

*I underestimated you.*
*I wanted to believe*
*you were containable*
*constrainable*
*and reliable*
*in the 'my way' kind of way.*
*The magician*
*hitman*
*slot machine*
*deal maker*
*earth shaker*
*genie-in-a-bottle*
*kind of way.*

*Then I recalled*
*that on a dark but necessary day*
*you took yourself*
*and my kind of way*
*and the cosmos*
*to a cross.*

*Then you went missing for three days.*
*And my world fell apart.*

*All my hope exhaled a forsaken surrender,*
*and my heart broke*
*and my dreams broke.*
*My kind of way*
*kind of died*
*again.*

*And there you were*
*alive and the same*
*but not really.*
*A resurrected form of you*
*that even took familiar friends*
*by surprise.*

*And that's what you keep doing.*
*To this day*
*you keep failing and disappointing me*
*in the best kind of ways.*

*Every time I think I've got you*
*where I think I need you*
*you disappoint and disappear*
*and turn up incognito*
*on a familiar path*
*at a regular meal*
*in an average garden*
*with a spark in your eye*
*that demands my attention.*
*You invite me again*
*to put my hand in your side*
*embrace you and kiss you*
*and get to know you again*
*in a new kind of way.*

*'Kind of Way'*
*David Tensen*
*The Wrestle (2020)*

So, am I saying here that alienation is possible? Yes and no. Yes, alienation is possible, in our minds and hearts. For reference, this 'kind of' separation (alienation) is addressed clearly in Colossians 1:21, Hebrews 9:9-14 and Ephesians 4:18. But friends, this separation is OUR doing. It is **us** who turn God into a hitmam, slot machine, deal maker, or genie-in-a-bottle. And it is the work of the Spirit to show us that there is no separation from Christ – not ontologically speaking. To summarise, the nature of our beings **is** in union with Christ, but the problem is, our hearts and minds create stories of separation. And this is an important point when it comes to this idea of decentering, because the first thing I think that we should consider decentering, is God. And by this, I mean the mental and emotional concepts and constructs of God that place us and God in separate fields of existence. Let me try and illustrate why this separation is problematic.

The thoughts I have of my wife Natalie are not actually Natalie. My own conscious constructs of my friend Gary are not Gary. Sure, my thoughts of both Natalie and Gary affect the relationship I have with them because I will treat them as I see them, but our thoughts of someone are not actually them. The nature of their being is not determined by my thoughts of them. In this same way, our thoughts of God, and our conscious constructs of God, are not God. This sounds obvious, but so many of us have been led to believe that our belief of God overrules and determines God's very being, along with God's unconditional love for us, and perhaps even salvation. Either we are in a mystical and ontological union with God in Christ or, somehow, we have gained the ability to think the truth of our being into a state of actual separation. If interpenetrative union with and in Christ is a non-negotiable given (as the early Church Fathers, Orthodox, Catholics, and many modern theologians suggest), then I think exploring how we mature within this divine union with Christ deserves consideration.

Decentric eldering starts with this simple and minimum truth: "You are not the center of the universe." This much we know from developmental psychology: Those who still think and behave like they are at the center of the universe are developmentally stuck in early childhood. The world needs more eccentric souls – and not just those who identify as Christian who spin around their notion of God. Let me unpack the idea of eccentricity, because it's an important concept in this book and the term decentric is a combination of the words decenter and eccentric.

By way of background on eccentricity, Christian psychologist and author Richard Beck, whom I admire greatly, wrote a series of blogs in 2014 on the topic of Eccentric Christianity. These thoughts also appear in his book, The Slavery of Death (2013). Beck openly confesses that he is using the work of David H. Kelsey who wrote about eccentric existence. Beck's work focuces on Christian Identity and the biblical call to be a peculiar people. I realise the term 'Christian identity' may be new to some readers, but it simply explains how a person understands and expresses their faith in Jesus Christ and how it shapes their life, values, and actions around that faith commitment. We put this to words quite often when we attempt to finish sentences like, "I'm a Christian, so…"

The word "eccentric" originally meant "out of center" in Greek (ek = out of, kentron = center). Interestingly, it was first used in astronomy to describe systems where Earth wasn't at the center. Today, we take for granted that the Sun, not Earth, is at the center of the solar system, but it was Copernicus' revolutionary model that suggested this was true. Before this, many Europeans assumed they were the center of the cosmos. Isn't maturity and science wonderful!?

David H. Kelsey uses this astronomical meaning as a metaphor for Christian spiritual growth: Just as the Earth was moved from the center in Copernicus' model, a Christian's identity involves moving their ego from the center of their life to let God be the central focus instead. In this model, the self orbits around God rather than expecting God to orbit around the self. This results in us being off-center or out-of-center: eccentric.

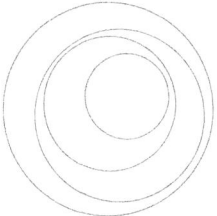

Eccentric Circles

I believe that living in the outer circles, off-center, is essential for a healthy and sustainable existence. Being off-center is also an essential step in healing and recovery. For example, most 12-step recovery programs, like Alcoholics Anonymous, have within them rules or tenets that a proposed Higher Power be leaned upon and surrendered to. They are encouraged to relinquish the personal role of *controller of all things*. It would seem that knowing you are not God, not in control, and not to be totally blamed (or praised) for things that happen around you is great for your mental health too.

All that said, I think that Richard Beck's suggestion to put God in the center and have an eccentric identity has, within it, a dynamic that may not have been considered or examined. And this is really important to consider, particularly when it comes to the idea of decentering everything, including God.

Reader: This may be a new and possibly blasphemous consideration, so please chew the following slowly.

If the God of the Christian faith is in fact composed of God the Father, God the Son, and God the Holy Spirit, then we should perhaps consider how they exist as three-in-one. Although not widely known, one of the most popular forms the Trinity has been described to exist in is a *circle dance*, or in theological terms, a 'perichoresis'. 'Peri' meaning round, and 'choresis' as in dance. (Think of the words periscope and choreography.) As touched on earlier, this more Orthodox and ontological view proposes a kind of mutual indwelling and interpenetration of the Father, Son, and Spirit. I won't spend too much time unpacking the significance of the perichoresis but do recommend theologian C. Baxter Kruger's work and writings, along with Richard Rohr's accessible book, The Divine Dance. Suffice to say, the idea of God being a circle dance has endured around 1,500 years of Christian thought.

You will likely have seen Perichoresis (or Circumincessio in Latin) symbolism around. Sometimes it looks like three people holding hands, dancing in a circle. It is also symbolised in the Trinity knot, which looks rather Celtic by nature. Regardless of how it is symbolised the question I would ask you is, 'What is at the center of the Trinity? If we simply look at popular trinitarian symbols and icons, nothing is at the center. There is always an empty space.

Celtic Triquetra (Trinity Knot)

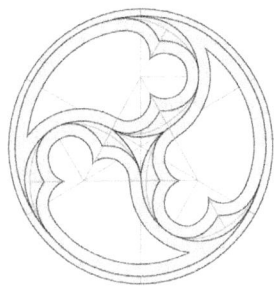

Gothic Triskele (window element)

Over my 30 years in church services, I have seen, from the pulpit, well-meaning pastors and preachers attempt to explain how the Trinity works. They proceed to bring three people up on stage from the audience, ask them to hold hands in a circle, perhaps dance around – then, they ask the congregation, 'Where are you in this Trinitarian picture?' On more than one occasion I have seen a preacher take somebody else from the audience and position them in the middle of the circle and have 'God' dance around them. They then explain that YOU and I are in the center of the Trinity. This may be done in innocence (or ignorance) because we **are** wrapped up in God's loving embrace, but I think the demonstration largely points towards the human-centric (anthropocentric) and egocentric tendencies that we desperately need to move away from. Theologically speaking, we are all in Christ, who is in the Trinity – so although we are caught up in Christ, we can't be the central most important axis God spins around. Instead, we exist on the circumference of the circle, decentered in mysterious union with Christ.

To repeat, we are not at the center of the Trinity. So, what, or who is? I would argue that nothing, NO THING, is at the center of the Trinity, and that might be some really good news.

I understand that divine spherical imagery may be a new concept to some readers, but I promise you, I am not the first to consider God in this spherical and containing way.

In the 12th century, Hermes Trismegistus proposed, "God is an infinite sphere, the center of which is everywhere, the circumference nowhere." (Book of the 24 Philosophers).

Also in the 12th century, poet and theologian Alain of Lille wrote, "God is an intelligible sphere, whose center is everywhere, and whose circumference is nowhere."

French mathematician, physicist, inventor, philosopher, and Catholic writer Blaise Pascal said: "The whole visible world is only an imperceptible atom in the ample bosom of nature. No idea approaches it. We may enlarge our conceptions beyond all imaginable space; we only produce atoms in comparison with the reality of things. It is an infinite sphere, the center of which is everywhere, the circumference nowhere. In short, it is the greatest sensible mark of the almighty power of God that imagination loses itself in that thought."

These are majestic and overwhelming thoughts, right? The absolute vastness and mystery of God should, as it did for Pascal, bring us to a point of lost thought. But how often does it? Instead, we are people obsessed with certainty, knowing, and explaining God through clever speech and prose. I would argue we should attempt to steer away from this kind of vain certainty. Again, our mind and conscious mind create the illusion of separation from God. Is it a surprise Jesus was crucified at Golgotha? Golgotha means 'place of the skull'.

To summarise, I am suggesting that from a Trinitarian perspective nothing belongs in the middle of God. The great philosophers I quoted similarly propose a paradox that 'everywhere' exists in the center of God (e.g. all things are held in God) but also that God has no circumference, no outer limit. Again, this may sound like a radical idea when compared to the ego-friendly God often portrayed within Western Christian consumerist constructs. It might even sound heretical when held against the popular dogma that God belongs at the center of our life. I would argue that most people who demand God be central are very quick to tell you that their construct, opinion, thoughts, and religious views of God are the correct one to centralise. Unfortunately, this centralising approach robs God of God's 'otherness' and binds us. We fail to see Christ incognito, on a familiar path, at a regular meal, in an average garden.

Beholding the otherness of God is one of the beautiful aspects of apophatic prayer practices like the ironically named 'Centering Prayer' practice taught by Fr. Thomas Keating, Cynthia Bourgeault, and others. These practices of prayer invite us to empty the mind of words and ideas of all things, including images and ideas of God, so that God will come to us as God's present self – not within the confines of our limited definitions of God. For Christians who, like me, were led to believe emptying your mind like this is dangerous and makes room for the devil, I see and understand your apprehension and fear – but I would challenge to you to not be afraid and learn to trust and see that God is magnificently bigger than you ever imagined. While we are discussing ingrained religious fears, I suspect some readers may be concerned that saying *all creation* is in mystical union with Christ sounds like pantheism. Pantheism suggests that created things like a tree or a dog ARE God. If you feel this way then I invite you to look into panentheism. This view holds the belief that God is greater than the universe and includes and interpenetrates it.

So, if this idea of decentering all things, including our concepts of God, is still difficult to think about, let me offer you an illustration through a story.

Imagine a person you are very fond of inviting you to join them for dinner at a restaurant which you have heard raving reviews about. You look forward to the event because you know this person sees you through the eyes of love. They get you. They are deep listeners. They are always thrilled to be with you and there is a great sense of belonging and possibility that accompanies being with them.

You haven't seen them for a while, so you get dressed as best you can. You arrive at the restaurant to find them waiting in the lobby. Gentle music is playing in the background, along with the quiet hum of intimate conversation between other couples. Your friend smiles and gives you a deep hug. You melt into their embrace and they into yours. You walk to the waiter who ushers you to your table. There is a lovely table for two tucked away in the corner. All things are perfect.

The waiter pulls back your seat and invites you to sit down and does the same for your friend. You take a seat at the table and there is a giant fresh bouquet of exquisite flowers sitting in a glorious vase set in the middle of the table. You spend some time discussing it's beauty and fragrance but you also notice you can't really see each other's faces beyond the flowers.

There is room to move the vase out of the way to the edge of the table, but as you go to carefully it, you notice it's not shifting. Your friend laughs and also tries to move the vase and notices the very same thing. You both look closely and notice that the vase has been attached to the center of the table, through the tablecloth, somehow.

You look around. Some tables have a vase in the middle. Couples are awkwardly trying to see around the bouquets. Some couples, it seems, have given up the battle with the flowers and are just eating in silence or are on their cell phones.

Looking again, you notice a small number of couples have vases that they have moved to the edge of their tables. And they are deep in face-to-face conversation. You and your partner agree that there is something beautiful at the center of your table and no one would deny that a stunning bouquet of flowers does not belong in a setting like this. But being fixed in the middle of the table hinders you from seeing the other – except through its foliage.

You signal to the waiter and explain that your vase is glued to the table. The waiter replies, "Yes, it is. This vase is fixed in the center." Then smiles and continues in a warm tone, "We do have a table nearby where the vase is *de*-centered and can be moved. Would you like that table?"

Without hesitation you both say yes. Not because you don't love flowers. You know flowers will still exist on the table being offered. But you say yes because the flowers are not in the center. Decentering the flowers makes room for the loving gaze and deep listening you have both been longing for.

If we center our image of God, even if our image seems as beautiful and inviting as a fragrant bouquet, it hinders our ability to see and connect with others. I suspect this is why there is *no thing* in the middle of the Trinity too, so that a loving gaze can cross the void, the Father to the Son, the Son to the Spirit, Spirit to the Father, and so on. The Good News is, we are caught up in this loving gaze, in union with Christ the Son. This loving gaze across this divine circle dance offers us a deep and necessary experience of intimacy (or in-to-me-see).

Metaphorically speaking, when you have something centered on the table of your life, as important, beautiful and wonderful as it may seem, including an imagined construct and idea of God, you hinder loving gaze and stunt relational opportunity for growth. Unless you learn to decenter everything, you must always look through the foliage and composition of things you have centered. You can't smell the other person because all you smell is flowers. You can't really see the other person as they are because you're seeing them through flowers.

Having said that, I am not advocating that decentering everything means we will see all things 100% clearly because decentering is a life-long practice and posture.

Becoming like God (theosis) is a process. However, I think it is possible to see more things clearly and be seen more clearly by others. The dim-seeing we all suffer from, to a degree, seems true of the life that we all live. Scripture tells us that we see as if in a mirror dimly (1 Corin 13:12). Ironically, this commonly repeated verse follows a verse calling the reader to maturity. "When I was a child, I spoke like a child, I thought like a child, I reasoned like a child. When I became a man, I gave up childish ways." (1 Corin 13:11). It may be fair to assume that seeing more clearly is a result of maturity in the ways of Love.

Now perhaps you're not comfortable with decentering God, and I respect that, that's your choice. You might not hold to a Trinitarian view of God; not every Christian does. You may never have thought or come across this ancient, seasoned term of God being like a circle dance. But I propose to you that decentering God allows God to be God and you to be in mystical truth-filled union in Christ and Christ in you. Together, as part of the circle, gazing lovingly upon everything that you see in heaven and earth - not being affected and influenced by a notion of God that a religious denomination nominated on your behalf. Because whatever you think of God, and however you paint God to be, not only says a lot about you, but deeply affects the way that you see others.

And so, for me, decentric eldering is an active and constant undoing of my idea, concept, and construct of God in ways that are untrue and do not bear good fruit in my life. This allows my worldview and Godview to evolve to a point where the lie of separation and alienation makes way for the truth that I am in union with God – who is the ultimate decentered circle. You and I are invited to join in this circle dance, this divine dance, this perichoresis with our everyday lives.

*Trinity is union.*
*A constant conversation.*
*A becoming belonging.*
*A covenantal choice.*
*A joyful expression.*

*Trinity is union.*
*A perichoresis of three.*
*A flow of oneness.*
*A convergence of rivers.*
*A swimmable source.*

*Trinity is union.*
*A bonded togetherness.*
*An eternal alarming reminder.*
*An invitation*
*to echo it's way*
*on earth*
*as it is in heaven.*

*'Trinity Is'*
*David Tensen*
*The Wrestle (2020)*

While we are speaking of the Trinity, there is one other lovely aspect of Trinitarian theology that is worthy of a few pages. This is the notion of 'kenosis'(self-emptying). Kenosis is a Greek term found in Philippians 2:6-7 which speaks of Christ as one "Who, being in very nature God, did not consider equality with God something to be used to his own advantage; rather, he made himself nothing (ekenōsen) by taking the very nature of a servant…"

This text from the New Testament describes Christ's self-emptying or self-humbling in the incarnation. However, the concept stretches beyond Christology and Trinitarian theology as a concept for spiritual formation. And I think it's a concept worth considering, especially within the practice of decentric eldering.

Highly regarded Swiss theologian and Catholic priest Hans Urs von Balthasar (1905-1988) suggests that "kenosis" as demonstrated within the Godhead (Trinity) underpins all subsequent kenosis. Balthasar suggested that Christ's self-emptying on earth as a servant was an extension or expression of the self-emptying nature of the Trinity. For the Father strips himself, without remainder, of his Godhead and hands it over to the Son; he 'imparts' to the Son all that is his."

Can you imagine a three-part adult relationship like a mother, father, and child where each party is dedicated to emptying themselves into one another? Imagine now that the transfer of power was transferred to one another through their hands and through a loving gaze. If these three people stood in a straight line, the person at one end would be full, and the other two empty. But in a circle with nothing in the middle, there is this constant flow of energy from one to another as every hand is held. An endless giving and receiving. If I were part of that kind of supply chain, I'd be dancing too. In fact, you and I are invited to say 'yes' to the reality of that divine dance of giving and receiving. This very basic explanation of 'kenosis' in the Trinity holds another key to decentric eldering.

Decentric elders have learnt the art of both self-emptying and have discovered a path to sustainable sources of divine supply. This supply source may look like many things. It might include reflective and relaxing activities such as contemplative prayer, reading, meditation, nature walks or time with animals. You might enjoy creative expressions such as journaling, music, the arts. For some it could be time with family, volunteering and community service, sports, or religious services. What we connect with may change with different seasons of life. A good question to ask ourselves often is, where do I feel deeply supported and replenished?

Decentric eldering, then, is marked by an accommodating approach to self-management. Not self-sacrifice, or self-beating, or self-hatred. Decentric elders simply don't burn out, they don't run themselves silly, they are not *noble martyrs,* and they don't blame others for 'making' them do things. They just keep travelling at an unapologetic pace which they gladly inhabit. There is an emptying out for others, but the source of their supply is at hand.

In 1997, world-famous saxophonist Kenny G set a world record by holding a single note without a break for 45 minutes and 47 seconds. He did this by employing a wind-instrument playing method called circular breathing. In circular breathing, a player almost empties their lungs, and while emptying the last bit of air from full cheeks, takes another breath in, creating a constant flow of air into the instrument. I've met a number of deeply spiritual people, including some Christians, who carry this deep, genuine, and authentic ability that enables them to pour into others and replenish simultaneously in a circular-breathing kind of way. Interestingly, so many of them carry a deep sense of **joy** that transcends happiness and produces a kind of strength and resilience in the pouring out. It's as if the loving gaze of the divine dance has been internalised and empowers them in a kenotic flow.

In summary, our mystical and ontological union with Christ in the Trinity offers us a picture of living a life that imitates God in a decentered and sustainable way – with nothing in the middle, not even a rigid and fixed image of God. This Trinitarian union of perichoresis, interpenetration, and kenosis encourages us to lovingly gaze upon each other, create belonging, and participate in the life-force and the life-flow of all living things.

Aside from decentering God in order to be in union with God, there is more to decenter if we want to reimagine eldering in our age. This includes our longing and demand to be heard in our later years, which we cover in the next chapter.

# Questions for reflection
# and discussion.

The chapter presents three perspectives on union with God (Covenantal/Forensic, Mystical/Ontological, and Existential/Relational). Which perspective resonates most with your spiritual journey? How might exploring different perspectives enrich our collective understanding?

How does the image of God as a "circle dance" (perichoresis) with nothing at the center compare with your own experience of the divine? What might we learn from this ancient understanding of the Trinity?

Consider the restaurant table metaphor with the flower vase. What beautiful things might we have placed at the center of our lives that inadvertently block our ability to truly see each other?

The concept of kenosis (self-emptying) is presented as central to both the Trinity and authentic eldering. Where have you witnessed this quality in elders you have known, and how might we cultivate it in ourselves?

"Whatever we think of God not only says a lot about us, but deeply affects how we see others." How have your images of God shaped the way you view and treat the people around you?

What does "circular breathing" look like in your spiritual practice? How might we develop sustainable sources of inner nourishment that allow us to give without becoming depleted?

What resistance do you feel to the idea of decentering God? What fears or hopes emerge when we consider moving our fixed concepts of God from the center of our tables?

# DECENTER BEING HEARD

*Perhaps humility feels like this:*
*to shut my mouth,*
*quiet my inner critique,*
*and make space for sapling and seed*
*only time away from tallness.*

*To leave generous gaps*
*in the canopy of wisdom.*
*To recall that I too*
*remain dependent*
*on the elements and shelter*
*of neighbours and strangers.*

*To live with a fragile knowing*
*that the unavoidable truth is*
*we all fall and break down*
*only to become a bed*
*for both friend and foe*
*to dig their own roots into,*
*just as we have done.*

*'Humility'*
*David Tensen (2024)*

Becca winced as her mother's voice carried across the retirement village cafe and she heard a phrase for what felt like the hundredth time that afternoon, "Well, when I was raising you children..." Becca, a young mother who had simply been trying to calm her restless toddler, now sat rigid. Her face a mask of polite endurance as her ageing mother launched into another detailed prescription for proper parenting.

Becca's mind wandered to a prior week, in a kind of contrasting hope. She was at a different café with her husband John where they both witnessed a precious sight at a nearby table. A lady in her eighties sat with a teenage girl, her granddaughter perhaps. What caught Becca and John's attention was the quality of their interaction. The senior lady wasn't speaking much at all, but her whole body was tuned to the girl's animated sharing. When the teenager paused, uncertain about something, the lady would offer a gentle "Tell me more about that..." The girl would lean in closer, her words flowing with increasing confidence. When the senior lady finally did share something from her own experience, the teenager listened with the same attention she had received.

The contrast was striking. Becca couldn't help but feel judged and defensive in her mother's presence. Her mother never stopped to enquire about her experiences and was always offering unsolicited advice on mothering, life, faith, cooking, and whatever the latest fear-inducing local news was broadcasting. In contrast, the older woman at the café created space for genuine connection and growth by focusing on understanding. Both older persons had something to share, but their approaches yielded vastly different results.

For several years, when I was a travelling teacher and healer of sorts, I would often introduce churches and organisations to a developmental model called The Life Model. It was developed by Dr Jim Wilder and others at a non-profit known today as Life Model Works. I remain a fan of their work and their simple-to-understand intergenerational maturity model which progressed through maturity tasks and phases from infant, to child, to adult, to parent, and then finally, elder. I reference their work throughout this book.

Whenever I introduced a group of people to the Life Model, I would highlight its list of proposed maturity tasks a person should have performed at each stage of life, up until the elder stage. When I got to the elder stage, without fail, I would get a good number of uncomfortable looks and responses.

The creators of the Life Model propose that true elders embody wisdom in their later years, after their last child turns 13 (or an equivalent age without children). In this model embodying wisdom comes through ones graceful acceptance of criticism or rejection, and ones courage to speak truth with love, even when faced with opposition. Elders serve without needing recognition but with a dedication to fostering growth and change, and genuinely delight in the success of the younger generation. Most of all, elders are committed to prioritising community well-being over personal interests.

You might have noticed there is nothing overt in that elder description about listening. This is because by elder stage good listening is a given. We should have learnt to good active listening way back before the parent stage, in the adult stage. The adult stage, according to their framework, is somewhere between 13 years old and the time you have your first child. The Life Model proposes that when someone fails to move beyond the adult maturity stage, your interactions with them will never feel truly mutual. You will go away feeling that in order to maintain a relationship with these stunted souls, you will always need to listen more, tolerate more, or give more, than they would ever be willing to do for you.

The ability to listen and consider another person is something we should start learning in our teen years, and this is really forged as we learn to take care of ourselves and a significant other (like a partner), simultaneously. This ability to bond within mutually satisfying relationships is something we are designed to get at home during infant and child stages. Yet, so many people do not experience this. Instead, traumatised, stressed, immature, and absent parents tend to replicate their own kind. And as we discussed in earlier chapters, many complex factors seem to have contributed to what has become the norm among many of our aged persons today; that being generations who do not have the capacity, skills, and ability to create adult relationships that are genuinely reciprocal. Sadly, very few older people ever developed the capacity to show equal interest in one another's lives and make space for others to appear and emerge **as they are** in this present moment. A decentric elder simply knows how and when to shut their mouths and also when to request a caring ear, without apology or coercion.

Perhaps this is a good time to mention that the Life Model is not the only developmental model to suggest that most people do not move beyond adolescence and early adulthood in the psycho-socio-spiritual sense. In Nature and the Soul (2019), Dr. Bill Plotkin presents an eight-stage developmental model called the Wheel of Life and argues that most people get stuck within consumeristic behaviours and never make it past stage 3 or 4 of the 8-stage wheel. Plotkin points out that our culture's arrested development at an adolescent stage creates widespread social dysfunction – from materialism and greed to hostility and discrimination. These destructive patterns aren't inherent to human nature, but rather emerge from an ego-driven society that hasn't matured into wisdom and interconnectedness with creation.

Whether it is the Life Model, the Wheel of Life, Carl Jung's stages of life, Jane Hardwicke Collings seasonal stages, Erick Erickson's psychosocial stages, Hagberg's Critical Journey, Robert Kegan's 5 stages – most psycho-socio-spiritual maturity models present a very similar and sobering reality of stunted development in our time. It was therefore no surprise that when I presented the Life Model maturity stages to a group of older persons, I would very often hear a kind of lament from those in the post-parenting season of life which sounded something like, "But David, no one listens to elders anymore." They'd continue, "The young people do not care that we have so much wisdom to share." There would be further comments that kids are rude, they are glued to their phones, and many more painful reasons that no one cares to hear from them. I respected and appreciated that they felt safe enough to voice this sense of loss, grief, and frustration.

However, this common lament reveals several things to me. Most importantly that many had mistaken 'older people' for 'elders', and as I am trying my darndest to point out in this book, an older person may be in an elder body, but this does not mean they inhabit or exhibit the psychological stage of a true elder. I didn't have succinct answers at the time, and because they were paying for my time, I dared not upset them too much. But here is how I might respond today: "Note how this complaint of young people not listening is really about **you**. The pain of feeling unheard also carries a hidden invitation to move beyond the need to be heard at all. Why? Because the practice of decentric eldering can be done in silence – in fact, I suggest deep listening is a hallmark of great elders; both human and more-than-human."

What do I mean by more-than-human? I mean other species that inhabit this glorious planet – of which we cannot live without. Consider, for a moment, the oak tree in autumn. It doesn't announce its offering of acorns to the forest floor. Equally, it doesn't grieve when squirrels take without acknowledgement. It doesn't keep a tally of which creatures benefit from its shade. The oak's wisdom lies in its silent giving, its unwitnessed generosity. Equally, consider the eldering power of wild oceans. These water bodies serve as a reminder that generous presence without words can give life and buoyancy to hungry mouths and heavy hearts. And what of the power of animals? When I bring our family dog 'Cosmo' into the aged care facility on my chaplaincy rounds, Cosmo says nothing – but his presence brings healing, joy, and fills the hearts of residents and staff. If you love elephants, you must find the story of conservationist Lawrence Anthony online. You'll read how, when Lawrence died, a herd of elephants he had saved on his reserve walked for 12 hours to his home to mourn his passing.

Flora and fauna aside, I think it is fair to confess that our yearning to be heard often masks a deeper attachment most of us have to significance. Some may argue this yearning is simply loneliness – but loneliness can't be cured with a monologue, can it? Too often, I think, people in their angst and insecurity are unconsciously desperate to remain the hero in (their) life's story. And because so many today have been the center-stage hero, victim, or martyr during the spring and summer seasons of their lives, this lament of "I have so much wisdom to offer" should not come as a surprise response among the ageing today. The ego we so carefully built over decades seems to cling desperately to importance and is willing to consume any ear that presents itself as a kind of pseudo-conversation. And I say pseudo-conversation because what many consider conversation today is, as poet John O'Donohue points out, simply an intersection of monologues - suggesting instead that when we truly converse, both parties are taken to a new place of knowing, together.

I believe that we cannot practise decentric eldering unless we acknowledge that being unheard comes to us as a kind of initiation, leading to the uncomfortable but necessary question: "What good am I, then?" This query must remain unanswered until it transforms into a more vital question: "What good can I call out in others?" This shift of questions mirrors the very practice of **blessing.** And I believe the current absence of blessing from authentic elders is nothing short of a heartfelt fracture in the spirit of the world today.

You may not know this, but the term 'blessing' in the Christian New Testament scriptures often appears as the translated term 'eulogia' in Greek. Can you see a familiar word there? Yes, eulogy - that kind word spoken over a dead person. A eulogy is an other-centric, gold-focused blessing spoken over another person. And somehow, this practice has been sequestered to a time when the person who may need to hear it with their living body cannot hear it. Blessing is a lost art in Western culture. I have taught about it over many years, across several countries, to thousands of people. And in all that time, I have never met anyone who isn`t drawn to the power of a spoken blessing, especially **from** an elder.

Now, you may be seeing a contradiction here. On one hand I am suggesting that being unheard is an invitation to grow. On the other hand, however, I am also suggesting that we should focus on imparting blessings. How do we bless if we aren't speaking? The answer to that is this: We must first master deep listening. Theodore Roosevelt has been attributed with saying, "No one cares how much you know, until they know how much you care." Isn't this what deep listening does? Doesn't it show that you care? And not just listening so that you can say your piece, but listening to really understand the other. I suggest that decentric elders who demonstrate maturity by 'listening to understand' are granted the opportunity to leave the earth having spoken life-giving blessings over every living thing – and it is their joy to do so.

It would be unfair for me to have this movement to deep listening sound like an easy intergenerational transition. Perhaps you have already learnt to listen deeply and are more like the grandmother in the café mentioned in the opening story. This doesn't mean that the world will listen. It certainly doesn't mean we will gain the attention of young people when we quiet ourselves and shut our mouths. With the introduction of social media, gaming, mass-streamed television, and increased multi-tasked work demands, people's attention spans have been dropping by the decade. Researcher Linda Stone calls this modern phenomena "continuous partial attention," and I don't think there is much that a person can do about this neurological shallow engagement except be available and demonstrate a state of being which many younger people long for; a settled presence that is thrilled to be with them.

I will expand on wisdom and knowledge in another chapter, suffice to say that wisdom emerges from a different place than knowledge. Decentric elders understand that wisdom emerges from making spaces for reflection, building a capacity to hold complexity, and sitting with uncertainty (to name a few). It may be true that today's mass media environment works against each of these elements, but this does not mean that people are not looking for deep wisdom and personal connection. The saying, "When the student is ready, the teacher will appear," seems to be true. You must learn to trust God to bring people to you who need your listening ear, settled presence, and perhaps some wisdom wrapped up in advice, a story, skill, or a question.

Like me, you might work in a job that requires a lot of listening. While authoring this book, my work as a part-time chaplain in aged care means I am basically paid to connect with, and listen to people for much of my work day. Some readers might think that sounds like a dream job. Other readers, I'm sure, think that listening all day might be akin to a slow death, of sorts. And I'm not going to lie, some days are very hard. Deep, attuned, and sincere listening can be draining. Good listening, not just waiting your turn to speak, takes time to develop. To decenter your response, your thoughts, your wanting to fix, correct, or retaliate takes time to develop. Any good listener has developed a skill made up of many micro skills. And if you don't think that good listeners are valuable, perhaps you haven't investigated the hourly rate of a good psychologist or counsellor.

There are volumes of books to read and courses to take to improve your listening skills. However, if you were to ask me how an authentic elder might both listen and respond, I think the Companioning framework is a great place to start. Alan D. Wolfelt, Ph.D., is the Founder and Director of the Center for Loss and Life Transition and creator of the companioning model. Although companioning is a model crafted to predominantly treat those grieving, mourning, and bereaved, I believe it offers us a perfect framework for decentric eldering. Largely because it decenters the listener as a kind of expert or fixer. Instead, it places the speaker and the listener alongside one another, on the edge of the circle, as companions. This is a subtle but significant shift in approach.

On the following pages are the eleven tenets of Companioning, according to Wolfelt from the book Companioning the Bereaved (2005). I suggest you read them slowly, and perhaps ask yourself if you have the capacity and ability to do this yet:

**Tenet One:**
Companioning is about being present to another person's pain; it is not about taking the pain away.

**Tenet Two:**
Companioning is about going to the wilderness of the soul with another human being; it is not about thinking you are responsible for finding the way out.

**Tenet Three:**
Companioning is about honouring the spirit; it is not about focusing on the intellect.

**Tenet Four:**
Companioning is about listening with the heart; it is not about analysing with the head.

**Tenet Five:**
Companioning is about bearing witness to the struggles of others; it is not about judging or directing those struggles.

**Tenet Six:**
Companioning is about walking alongside; it is not about leading.

**Tenet Seven:**
Companioning is about discovering the gifts of sacred silence; it does not mean filling up every moment with words.

**Tenet Eight:**
Companioning is about being still; it is not about frantic movement forward.

**Tenet Nine:**
Companioning is about respecting disorder and confusion; it is not about imposing order and logic.

**Tenet Ten:**
Companioning is about learning from others; it is not about teaching them.

**Tenet Eleven:**
Companioning is about compassionate curiosity; it is not about expertise.

Wolfelt's companioning model offers rich insight into how elders might reimagine their role. Rather than seeing ourselves as center-stage knowledge dispensers, we become wisdom holders who create space for others' understanding to emerge. Let's consider a few tenets that might be a good place to start when it comes to decentric eldering.

Being present to pain (Tenet 1), whether physical, emotional, or spiritual, often seeks acknowledgment more than answers. When elders can sit with others' struggles without rushing to fix or advise, they offer a rare and precious gift. This requires us to be comfortable with silence, have capacity to hold space for difficult emotions, and be able to trust in the healing power of witnessed experience. Being present to pain, particularly if you have similar unhealed and unprocessed pain in your own life, makes this a sincere challenge. I recall when I started learning inner healing modalities in my mid-thirties, it was a genuine struggle to be present to another's pain while mine was being triggered. It was so hard not to make it an 'OMG, me too' moment and derail the entire process.

Heart-centered listening (Tenet 4) moves us beyond intellectual engagement to heart-level presence. This means listeners learn to attend to emotional undertones, respond to the feelings beneath the words, and offer empathic resonance rather than solutions. Ironically, when an elder demonstrates heart-centered listening, they are largely practising a decentric practice of not fixing or intellectualising what the other is sharing. What so many people fail to understand is there is so much that can be healed and resolved with an attuned heart, a loving gaze, and gentle nods of understanding.

Offering the gift of sacred silence (Tenet 7) in a world of constant noise is another rare gift. This involves recognising that wisdom often emerges in the spaces between words, allowing pauses for integration and reflection, trusting that silence can be as nourishing as speech. Again, it is incredible how many people, across ages and genders, simply cannot shut their mouths and sit in silence with another. I believe that decentering from the urge to talk is a key for true eldering, especially when supporting those who are grieving.

Some may argue at this point that these 11 tenets, and the notion of companioning are only good for the grieving. I would suggest you listen for a moment to the conversations much of the world is having. And I don't mean pleasantries like, 'Nice weather we're having today', or 'How good was the game on the weekend!?'. If you actually listen, with your heart, to many deeper and serious conversations people have, so many are grief-filled and loss-laden. For example, where someone may share that their child is struggling to fit in at school. You could see that as a complaint, a whinge, unnecessary and unsolicited drama, or you might notice that beneath this is a kind of grief that the child they love isn't doing as well as they hoped. Perhaps there is a sense of loss they are feeling as a parent that they are powerless to change the circumstance. My editor, Rachel, who lives in Japan, has pointed out that the Japanese concept of **kuuki-wo-yomu** or "reading the atmosphere" is an important form of non-verbal communication. Because of the collective nature of their society, Japanese people have been socialised to pick up body language, tone and to try to read between the lines – tuning into a deeper sense of how the other person is feeling. I promise, if you learn to genuinely listen and read the atmosphere, you will hear grief and loss everywhere, even under masks of toxic positivity, anger, frustration, and seemingly petty complaints.

Before moving on from this topic, in 2025 I interviewed author and spiritual companion Felicia Murrell on my podcast to speak on companioning. Felicia has 4 adult children, in their late 20s onwards, and I asked her how companioning has informed her parenting. Here is a transcribed portion of what she said:

> One of the things that was important to me as the kids got older was to move from the parent-child hierarchy of "Mama tells you what to do, you do it, you don't have a say.", to "You are human, I'm a human. We're here to remove that sense of hierarchy so this is an equitable relationship."
>
> And one of the ways I had to do that was to say to my adult kids, "I want you to decide how much you are in a relationship with me and what that looks like. And it's not that I'm not going to show up for you. I will always do that. I'll always be present. But I don't want you to feel obligated just because we have this hierarchical kind of thing of, *I'm the parent, you're the child.* I want the relationship because you want it - and you need to decide what that looks like now as adults. So what does it now look like to be in an adult-to-adult relationship?"

Notice the language and posture someone takes in companioning. It's non-hierarchical. There is no coercion, control, or inequality. It's invitational. It's patient. It's equitable. It reminds me of the way the Trinity operates. No one or thing belongs in the middle. This meeting-as-equals is sadly missed in too many child-parent relationships where the children are now adults. Decentric elders make it easy for others to meet them in an adult-to-adult relationship. Like Felicia demonstrated, as parents of adult children we must work to lower ourselves from the old parent-over-child dynamic, and also encourage the child to move from the child-under-parent way of thinking. This is best done gradually. However, without intention or discussion we all tend to fall into old habits. This includes unhelpful habits of listening to our adult children as eternally responsible and rescuing parents. By the way, if you are asking when a child becomes a young adult, many cultures believe around age 13 is when this transition from childhood to adulthood begins. And in the absence of rites of passage events in the West, I believe we need to make it clear to our children that they are not just between stages (teen-age), but young adults. Given that this stage of adolescence is where many seem to get stuck in their psycho-socio-spiritual formation, companioning through listening and lifestyle across generations and genders seems more vital for our collective growth than ever.

It would seem that we are created for increased capacity for companioning. Research by Yorkston et al. (2010) suggests that the art of listening transforms as we age, but not in ways our youth-centered culture might expect. While our ears and eyes may need more support to track both sight and sound at once, something remarkable unfolds. Like master musicians who can hear the whole orchestra while playing their part, older adults (70+) often develop an intricate capacity to listen between the lines and catch the unspoken notes in a conversation. They might take longer to respond in fast-moving discussions, but this slower pace often carries deeper understanding. When supported by environments that honour this rhythm (good lighting, minimal background noise, unhurried conversation spaces) older adults demonstrate how physical changes can open doorways to deeper listening and understanding. What might appear as a limitation in older adults becomes an invitation to listen differently, to hear with the heart as much as the ears.

I spoke of archetypes and archetypal energy earlier in the book, of which there are many. There are three that come to mind which may help embody and exemplify what decentric eldering may look like, in light of this chapter: the witness, the companion, and the sacred fool. These archetypal patterns offer templates for how authentic elders might inhabit their role in ways that foster genuine connection and growth. By consciously drawing on these different modes of listening, elders can remain flexible and responsive to what each situation requires. There is plenty of information on these archetypes online (if you wish to do a deep-dive):

**The Witness** moves through our stories as one who holds space for transformation through their profound presence.

**The Companion** appears as those who walk alongside others in their growth, offering partnership rather than dominance.

**The Sacred Fool** teaches us that wisdom often wears unexpected masks of compassionate curiosity.

It would be fair to ask, again, how it is I am advocating that we decenter being heard but all the archetype examples above were spoken and listened to by someone (at some point). The concern that "being a good listener means being silent" is understandable, particularly for generations who grew up in environments where it was taught that children were to be "seen and not heard." Am I suggesting that post-parenting, we just shut up and remain in silence and only speak when spoken too? The fear that cultivating listening skills somehow diminishes one's voice or wisdom requires contextual consideration, especially in our new noisy mass media landscape. Let's consider what researchers are discovering.

Media scholar Marshall McLuhan observed that each new communication technology reshapes not just what we say, but how we listen and engage. Today's digital natives (those born after 1980) inhabit a world where information flows constantly and from multiple directions. This shift challenges traditional patterns of elder-to-younger communication, but it doesn't diminish the value of elder wisdom – it changes how that wisdom might best be shared.

In today's uncharted age, when something unsolicited or irrelevant comes our way, we can simply change channels on the remote, or move on to the next video, podcast or article with a tap of a screen. Theorist David Altheide points out that our new communication landscape has fundamentally altered social processes and relationships. Younger generations often process information collaboratively, through discussion and shared exploration rather than traditional top-down instruction. This shift doesn't mean elders should be silent; rather, it invites them to participate in more dynamic ways.

Researcher Walter Ong reminds us that oral cultures traditionally valued listening as much as speaking - it actually was print culture that began emphasising one-directional communication. Perhaps our digital age, despite its challenges, offers an opportunity to reclaim some of that balance. The goal isn't silencing older voices but amplifying their impact through deeper engagement.

It's important for us all to remember that true wisdom isn't diminished by listening – it's enhanced. As we develop listening skills, our moments of speaking often become more powerful, more targeted, and more transformative.

This intricate dance between listening and responding without overwhelming or hijacking a conversation is a fine skill to learn and maintain. Suffice to say that decentric eldering is not a practice of saying nothing at all. It is understanding that what you have to say, as wise, exciting, relevant, and interesting as it might be (to you), does not belong in the center of the circle. Those practising decentric eldering know very well that you cannot companion (verb) from the center of the circle.

Decentric elders know their voice is not the most important voice in the room. They understand that shallow intersections of monologues change very little. Decentric eldering, therefore, is a living demonstration of loving equity and equality towards all creation, including the more-than-human. It announces, by its attuned presence to the other, that they belong and everyone in the circle, including them, matters deeply.

# Questions for reflection
# and discussion.

What aspects of humility seem particularly important for eldering as you reflect on its nature and purpose?

What distinguishes an approach of giving unsolicited advice from one of primarily listening in intergenerational interactions? How have you experienced both approaches?

What might it mean to practise eldering "in silence"? Why is this challenging in a culture that values being heard?

Among the "Companioning" tenets presented, which resonates most strongly with you and why?

How might "being unheard" serve as an invitation to grow? How does this invitation challenge typical expectations about ageing and wisdom?

What connections do you see between "blessing" and the practice of decentering being heard?

What practical steps could you take to develop deeper listening skills as part of your own eldering practice?

# DECENTER KNOWING

In a brightly lit conference room in Melbourne, fifteen executives sat through their fourth leadership development workshop of the year. The facilitator, Taliah, projected her slides onto the wall, each bullet point offering another framework for "wisdom in leadership." The execs took notes on their laptops, adding to their growing collection of methodologies and models.

During the lunch break, Taliah watched as Aaron, a recently retired CEO turned consultant, pulled out a book titled "The Four Ladders to Wisdom." He'd highlighted many pages. "I've read nine books on wisdom this year," he told her proudly, "I'm becoming quite the expert."

The irony hung in the air between them. Here was wisdom, reduced to a commodity – something to be acquired through bullet points, relegated to rubrics, distributed in digital downloads. Wisdom, true wisdom, cannot afford to be swallowed up into the same soup as knowledge.

As it happens, I gained a Bachelor's degree in Organisational Leadership in my late 30s and later conducted research around Change Management practices in a healthcare setting for my Honours degree. I then spent four years consulting in a leadership development and pastoral care role at a large multinational charity. This much has become clear; the LeaderShip is a noisy ship to be on – far noisier than the FollowShip or the ElderShip. Being a subject matter expert on leadership is very 'in vogue', and I suspect it's largely because we assume big corporations will pay handsomely for training and tools, but also because the ego loves the idea that it is leading leaders. There are hundreds of thousands of books on the topic of leadership, along with countless leadership seminars, coaches, programs, podcasts, and videos. Among titles and topics, you will see the terms 'knowledge' and 'wisdom' thrown around as if they were synonyms. But they are not the same, and I would suggest that those practising decentric eldering understand this difference.

Unsurprisingly, many of us have mistaken knowledge for wisdom. The line between the two has become incredibly blurry. Many of us would struggle to explain the difference between the two. To be honest, I find it a challenge to write about because explaining wisdom requires an amount of knowledge. In other words, to point out what wisdom is, you have to know what it is, or who it is, or how it's embodied and demonstrated. To avoid sounding pithy or cliché I want to draw from some academic work around wisdom - knowing that others before me have spent countless hours reading and synthesising work around wisdom.

To narrow the context, I'm leaning toward academic literature that equates wisdom with ageing. Firstly, let's consider a summarised definition of wisdom by Parisi et. al (2009).

*Wisdom encompasses the integration of cognitive, personality, affective, experiential, and social dimensions, highlighting its multidimensional complexity. This construct appears modifiable, suggesting certain contexts may nurture wisdom's development throughout the lifespan.*

In other words, wisdom refuses simple categorisation. It combines domains of knowledge, experience, and capability into a kind of circle-dance of its own which transcends any single environment or aspect of human functioning. And if it isn't clear by now, let me say (along with others) that wisdom does not arrive as ageing's consolation prize. The later years of life offer no guarantee of wisdom's flowering.

As we age, it is true that we gather knowledge from life's harsh and beautiful lessons, but wisdom asks more of us than mere accumulation of knowledge – and certainly much more than the accumulation of facts, data, and information. Wisdom demands we metabolise both positive and negative experiences, allowing them to transform us rather than simply inform us. And it should be said that wisdom speaks through the body and heart as much as through the mind. It seems true that those walking wisdom's path develop an inhabited sensitivity to their own and others' suffering and joy. Yes, this means that becoming wise includes cultivating emotional literacy - reading the language of feelings with nuance and responding with attunement rather than reaction. You might notice that the invitation to decenter being heard (in the previous chapter) and decenter being knowledgeable (in this chapter) cannot be easily separated.

Decentric elders understand that being heard and having knowledge are important, but they **decenter their own need to be center-stage distributors of things they know**. They push themselves, and everything else, to the edge of the circle. They make sure no thing and no person is in the middle. Decentric elders create space and time for others, and themselves, to synthesise knowledge, experiences, and capabilities. Decentric elders, therefore, become very skilled at spotting desperate measures that they, and others, take, in selling cheap facts and irrelevant data as kinds of synthesised pseudo-wisdom.

Spotting the difference between knowledge and wisdom takes time. I would argue that the difference is felt in the whole person, as much as it is acknowledged cognitively. We tend to treat knowledge much like we store books on shelves, linen in cupboards, and tools in sheds. Wisdom, on the other hand, is **inhabited** like a favourite reading chair, the embrace of a faithful friend, or quiet reflection.

Wisdom comes in slowly, honouring stillness and deep breaths.
Knowledge rushes to fill silent spaces.

Wisdom arrives as a thought to be considered.
Knowledge appears as a fact to be accepted.

Wisdom bubbles up from soft bellies burdened by love, and foot pads calloused from trials.
Knowledge travels short distances on electrical currents just centimetres from the mouth, with efficiency.

Wisdom may sound like uncertain answers to questions.
Knowledge seems to know without really knowing.

Wisdom builds blurry connections and doors that open to wonder.
Knowledge builds walls and gates guarded by limitations and insecurity.

Several years ago, after pouring out my heart to a man I considered an elder in my life, some of the most profound advice he ever gave me sounded like, "Hmmm. There is no easy fix to that problem. That's hard, David." Here was a man who was decades older than me, with troves of knowledge, experience, and capability at his disposal, letting me know I was not alone in the complexity of my position. It wasn't a young peer saying, "I Dunno!". It was not an expert giving me four things I could try in order to resolve things. It was not a codependent parent or spouse unable to sit with me in my suffering, wanting to rescue me like I was a 6-year-old who forgot their school lunch. Instead, it was a person who decentered their internalised database and assured me that what I was experiencing was surely difficult.

I am not discounting knowledge or being heard. I am arguing that they don't belong in the middle of decentric elders. In fact, it would seem that decentric elders have much to say about all they know. Most have great knowledge, experience, and capacity. However, the very act of decentering their need to share knowledge and be heard, gives them a kind of gravitas and presence that is best described as wisdom.

When it comes to spiritual, religious, and holy matters, this kind of wise presence is also felt by the discerning heart. As someone who has spent nearly three decades around theological literature and discussions, I have come to a point now where so much of this knowledge of God has had to make way for mystery, morph into uncertainty, and decenter itself into open wonder. God, it seems, was too much for my soul in the first half of life, so I held what I could in knowledge. Recently, while meditating on this gradual transition, I wrote this poem:

A poet once proclaimed
that the idea of God
was too much
for the young to grasp,

that they were lacking
days lived
or dreams lost
to carry the concept
of a divine being,

that the immature
were more likely to mistake
certainty for truth
and that truth for a faith
  that God would bend for.

Now, I am slowly seeing
the wisdom of reserving
sacred speech
and steeped silence
for life's second half,
finding myself less interested
in being right about God
and increasingly at peace
with the way life
presents itself;
that being,
a bittersweet ballad
of everything's longing
to belong.

*It would also seem*
*that well-worn eyes*
*are better at seeing*
*God's outstretched arms*
*hold all these longings together,*
*with love.*

*'Longing'*
*David Tensen (2024)*

There are certain portions of my poems I carry in my bones. The line in this poem "life is… a bittersweet ballad of everything's longing to belong." is one of those portions. When I spend time with older people, who by all accounts of age should be well into eldering, yet are still stuck and centered on regurgitating knowledge and data about all kinds of unsolicited things, I recite this line to myself. Everything longs to belong. I then ask myself if I can hold space for this soul needing to be seen, heard, affirmed and legitimised. This can surely be a test – particularly if your job requires you to spend significant time with the aged and you are often many decades younger than them. Perhaps it's dishonouring, but in order to cope and hold space for them, I sometimes imagine them as adolescent and young adults. I think about the young people in the 101 classes I teach at university. I notice the same interplay between them all – a built-in posturing among peers fuelled by a longing to belong. I recall 1 Corinthians 8:1 "Knowledge puffs up, but love builds up." I remind myself that most of the Silent and Boomer generations endured wars, depressions, and grew up elderless – absent of wisdom transmission. I remind myself how lonely many are, and **how far I still have to go.**

I have used the term 'wisdom transmission' a number of times already in this book, particularly in the opening chapters. It is a term used commonly among people who write about eldering and development from a multigenerational standpoint, so I think it's best to explain why wisdom is something that is transmitted.

In a society shaped by data retention and recall, we find ourselves starved of true wisdom transmission. Many have come to simply accept that, like Aaron in the opening leadership training story, we can gain, retain and regurgitate wisdom like a tool, of sorts. I hope that it is clear to you now that wisdom and knowledge are not interchangeable. Wisdom may well contain knowledge, but it is far more subjective and integrated than knowledge. In fact, we might even say that wisdom is an integrated form of knowledge. Therefore, the psychological conditions for wisdom to be both transmitted and received require far more than bullet points and frameworks. What I'm about to describe forms part of the boned skeleton upon which decentric eldering hangs its flesh.

For wisdom to flow from elder to community, the elder must first undergo a radical psychological reorientation. This isn't about accumulating enough years or reading enough books to become "quite the expert." Instead, as most developmental frameworks will prescribe, the elder must move far beyond ego-driven concerns and personal agendas. This includes the need to be seen as wise.

The decentric elder has integrated their whole life, with all its imperfections, failings, and shadows into the circle. They inhabit their being and their becoming. These elders are capable of transmitting wisdom by having cultivated what might be called psychological spaciousness - the capacity to hold complexity without reducing it to simple formulas or tidy solutions. They are, as mentioned earlier in the book, fat and generous souls.

Those receiving wisdom require their own psychological readiness. You cannot download wisdom like a software update. The receiver must be developmentally positioned to accommodate and embody what is offered. Consider how readily we dismiss wisdom when we haven't yet lived enough to recognise its truth. The posture needed is one of openness without idealisation. If we place elders on pedestals, much like the distance people create with their deities, we introduce an unnecessary distance that inhibits true transmission. (Again, a good case for eldering as companioning.) Instead, wisdom reception blooms in critical engagement. Wisdom is transferred by actively processing rather than passively accepting. Yes, it takes varied levels of emotional maturity to handle wisdom that may challenge our existing worldviews or identities. This tension is often needed. Decentric elders act out of love, but that does not mean that they are always nice or agreeable folk. As my poem states, the young are more likely to mistake certainty for truth and that truth for a faith that God would bend for. This kind of naivety is normal in the juvenile mind, but is unbecoming in elders who are practised at letting go.

Wisdom transmission may also fail when we confuse wisdom with being clever or right. Decentric elders understand that inhabiting uncertainty often characterises wisdom more authentically than certainty does. The psychological condition here involves tolerance for ambiguity and paradox. Where the immature mind seeks definitive answers, the mature heart has developed capacity for holding opposing truths simultaneously – even unpopular ones. Personally, I find the wisdom of loving your enemies to be a great example of this paradoxical wisdom. For decades I treated this saying of Jesus as a command to white-knuckle through. It would be far easier to go with the black and white version of loving my neighbour (allies) but hating my enemies. Here is the whole verse, note the simple and definitive reasonable commands that Jesus pushes against, paradoxically.

Matthew 5:43-45 "You have heard that it was said, 'You shall love your neighbour and hate your enemy.' 44 But I say to you, love your enemies, bless those who curse you, do good to those who hate you, and pray for those who spitefully use you and persecute you, 45 that you may be sons of your Father in heaven; for He makes His sun rise on the evil and on the good, and sends rain on the just and on the unjust."

Loving one's enemies, doing good to them, blessing and praying for them is not only very difficult, but largely unreasonable and unpopular. We continue to live in a world which rewards and fuels emotionally charged conflict. For example, social media algorithms are coded to promote posts that stir hatred and strong emotions. The evening TV news channels highlight stirring stories much the same, as do newspapers and basically any media outlet that is bent on keeping us in states of heightened engagement. Why? Mainly because their business models are advertisement-based. How utterly destructive it would be if we all woke up to the wisdom of elders and sages by loving and praying for our enemies. How depleted of power would our immature world-leaders be if everyone, including their followers loved their enemies? On love, Stanford social theorist René Girard (1923-2015) wrote, "If all men loved their enemies, there would be no more enemies". Yes, there would be no more enemies.

Which leads us back to decentric eldering and the call for us to decenter knowledge (which puffs up, interrupts wisdom transmission, creates enemies, and perpetuates itself throughout generations). If you feel the pull towards decentric eldering, you must consider the place of knowledge in your life. I would suggest it not only needs to be decentered but also transformed, along with experience and capacity, into a wisdom that creates the kind of belonging that all creation yearns for.

To those who are well into life's second half, it may be time to decenter the decades of experience, accomplishments, and hard-won expertise that has got you this far. I'm not saying it is invalid; it simply doesn't need to belong in the middle. The inner expert must resign their post and enter the larger fold – where true communion is found. It is time to move from being a knowledge-dispenser to a wisdom-holder. It may also be time to move from selling certainty to your anxious self (and others), to inhabiting the great uncertainty and wonder that accompanies wisdom but embodies and transmits a peace that transcends understanding.

To finish this chapter on knowledge, and keeping in mind the prior chapter on listening, I'd like to recommend a simple and powerful exercise that I heard poet David Whyte once present. It has been an exercise Natalie and I have done on occasions. It was often confronting and has revealed things we had each been blindly centering in our lives. The exercise is this: ask someone close to you, family or friend, if there is a conversation you need to stop having. And when I say conversation, I simply mean, "What do I need to stop talking about in the same way, and as often?" Many things we call conversations are unresolved wounds, loss, and disappointment which deserve to be decentered. Again, not because they are unimportant, but because they deserve integration, not segregation. I remember asking Natalie about this and she said, "You need to stop talking about our bankruptcy.". In 2013 we (technically me) went into voluntary bankruptcy over $45,000 of personal debt we simply could not pay back. The story is complex but since that event I had done a lot of inner work to reconcile what had happened because I felt such shame as a husband, father and provider. However, I kept bringing it up as a kind of hero story where I'd fought the dragon, got beaten, lost my ability to walk upright, but managed to leave the battle with my life, albeit with a limp and scarring.

Natalie was right. I had been centering the story for unhealthy attention and it was a conversation I now needed to stop having with myself and others.

So, what about you? What conversation do you need to decenter? What knowledge needs to make room for wisdom?

# Questions for reflection and discussion.

How might you articulate the distinction between knowledge and wisdom based on your own experiences?

When have you observed that "knowledge puffs up, but love builds up" in your own life or community?

How does wisdom transmission differ from knowledge transfer in your experience?

When has uncertainty led to greater wisdom in your experience? How might "inhabiting uncertainty" characterise wisdom more authentically than certainty?

What makes wisdom like "love your enemies" difficult to embody in today's polarised culture? How might you approach such paradoxical wisdom?

How might the perspective that "life is... a bittersweet ballad of everything's longing to belong" relate to wisdom in your own life?

What conversations might you need to stop having or decenter in your own life? What might make these conversations difficult to release?

# DECENTER DEATH

I believe most parents will agree that regardless of how much knowledge and theory they gained before their parenting journey, the praxis, the practicality, and the outworking of being a parent were largely developed during the parenting process. We learn by doing because effective parenting is both a process and a practice. Of course, the gaining of the knowledge, the application of theory, and preparation for the season ahead all help too.

I still have a photo of myself with my two-month-old daughter on my lap, sitting on a couch, reading a book on parenting babies. I was 26 and quickly realising that my child was unlike the 'clockwork and compliant' little human many books (at the time) described. The promises of the calm and compliant infant didn't seem to matter to my child. As my two sons entered the world, it became very obvious that parenting is as unique as every person. It is a lengthy work that creates opportunities for little persons to know who 'they' are, while simultaneously creating opportunities for parents to move further into a kind of paradoxical knowing through self-forgetting.

True of any decade, there are parents who believe that their very own parents (often their mother), sacrificed 'too much' of herself for her kids. It is common to hear people say their mother '...did not take care of herself ', was '...an embarrassment around friends', and '…really just poured too much of her life into her children'. They might say that about their fathers too - that '…he worked so hard for us' and '...didn't do much for himself'. Ironically, there are parentless children and children with self-absorbed and dysfunctional parents, who would give the world to have a parent who is present, gives, sacrifices, puts themselves last, and does what is needed to provide a loving and safe home for their children. This much we know, someone always pays for the posture of the selfish parent or a self-absorbed parent - first the children, then the community, because this parent often stays developmentally stuck, all the way to the grave. Personally, I don't think we can afford more eternally unsatisfied and over-entitled consumers.

Even though this may be unpopular in the midst of a self-care, self-help zeitgeist, I believe that parenting is a decades-long process. It is an invitation to become others-focused - an apprenticeship in self-forgetting, selflessness, kenosis, and selective self-management. And please hear me, I am not advocating for self-abandonment, martyrdom, co-dependency, or enmeshment here – these behaviours are as damaging as their counterparts.

Also, before I get warranted emails and comments from those who, for whatever reason, are without children (at an age they could be), I would propose that we have a planet full of humans, and more-than-human beings, who need some kind of sacrificial caregiving – whether that be the poor, sick, infants, disabled, animals, or habitat. I suggest that there are very few reasons that most cannot empty themselves into others, in some way, they want.

And so, I (and others) propose that the journey towards effective eldering is a maturity-focused progression of sustained parenting and caregiving. This progression requires a wider and wiser kind of self-forgetting, self-emptying, and joyful dying to one's sense of importance and subsequent ego-centricity. Eldering is, if entered into and practiced consciously, an invitation into a soul-expanded awakening in, as the poet Rumi put it, a "dying before we die". Yes, I have gone from parenting to death. And why not, we were created by two people and we are all destined to die. These are the inevitable bookends of life. Are you uncomfortable with talking about death? You're not alone.

In the 1970s, American cultural anthropologist Ernest Becker suggested that the great "denial of death" is upon us in the West. It seems we have successfully sanitised and removed ourselves from seeing, hearing, and smelling death. When was the last time you witnessed the death of the sentient animals you may consume? Unless you are a hunter, a conscious vegetarian, or an ethical vegan, my guess is that you have given little thought to the livestock (now deadstock) you purchase, which has been murdered, butchered, and nicely packaged in sterile containers at your local supermarket. And why should you? All that uncomfortable stuff happens out of view, reinforcing our denial of death and saving us from an uncomfortable reality. Should it be a surprise then that we rarely even like to speak of our own death with a sense of honesty? Most prefer to believe death isn't real. Yet, as a palliative nurse recently reminded me, "Death is one of the most real moments of your life.".

We have even removed death from our vocabulary. Did you know that the 'living room' in your home was once called 'the parlour' or 'receiving room'? As funeral parlours became a commercial phenomenon last century, and the dead were moved out of the home, the parlour became a 'living room'. Yes, we successfully outsourced another confronting reminder of death – along with animal slaughter and the dying-aged. And for some reason, most of us still enjoy seeing death and violence as forms of entertainment on our screens, whether it be in film or games. I'm not sure why this is. Is it because we are comfortably distanced from death? Is it because we somehow see death coming to insignificant and 'bad' people who we don't know, while secretly convincing ourselves that we are not like them?

Western culture's tragic denial of death is one reason most people struggle to accept their inevitable demise. Another is that many haven't experienced the conscious sense of dying to self, including the ego they carefully constructed during the first half of life. Why are we so incredibly reluctant to inhabit both the age we are and the age we live in? The lack of effective and authentic eldering across the West has certainly not helped.

To clarify, this overly common kind of death-denying pseudo-eldering I am wanting to challenge in this book has, in psychological terms, contributed to the vast kind of 'arrested development' in our culture today. I'd like to suggest that we are here, and headed for a kind of sad and stagnant repeat of this in society today because many are not willing to embrace the post-parenting, second-half, autumn-and-winter seasons of life. Why? Because it leads towards our end, our unimportance, our demise, and a possible messy ending. Those who work in aged care, hospice, or among the dying, (as I do), know what this looks like. We hear death, smell death, and witness it daily. Please, let this truth settle into your soul - no one is exempt from death and dying.

Why does this all matter: the dying before we die, the sacrificial caregiving, the exposure to death, the acceptance of our fragility as a species? Well, to many people, it won't matter because they continue to mistake having more, or doing more, for **being more.** They violently defend their own right to do as they see fit, and tend to be in shock and disbelief when troubles and grief find them or their community. To many, speaking of death is too heavy, too morbid, too much. Even many religious folk would rather subscribe to an individualistic salvation ideology that reads more like the legal 'terms and conditions' section of an eternal insurance policy than face the existential angst that drives many of them to defend their doctrine with utter meanness, violence, and plain stupidity.

But among the masses, there are those who quietly and genuinely know that the practice of decentering all things that demand center place in our hearts – whether it be our health, wealth, success, fame, addiction, family, failings, religious devotion and anything else – is paramount to walking out the last decades of their life in beauty, joy, and truth. These decentric elders understand, with all their being that, "Seeing the end of your life is the birth of your ability to love being alive. It is the cradle of your love of life." (Stephen Jenkinson, Die Wise, 2015).

I spoke of gerotranscendence in an earlier chapter. To recap: Gerotranscendence is a developmental theory about ageing. It proposes that as people age, they transition from a materialistic and rational view of life to a more cosmic and transcendent view. This shift leads to greater life satisfaction, self-acceptance, and redefined relationship with time, space, life and death. Some researchers suggest one in five Westerners will experience gerotranscendence in their later years. This gift generally comes to those who make room for death and accept that it is coming. They welcome it into the circle of their life. Not as centered, not expelled, not ignored, but on the edge, with everything else that belongs. Those fighting death, fearing death, and denying death's existence are rarely gifted the experience of gerotranscendence. I would suggest that decentering death, as a focal point to either be feared, endured, or enjoyed, is a necessary part of decentric eldering. And I would also add that excluding it from the circle of your life altogether is not possible. Ignoring death and pretending it won`t happen to you, or those you care about, is another form of denial disguised as bravery or stoicism. In reality, this culture-supported ignorance is an immature, dangerous self-deception that is psychologically tiring for those around you, because time waits for no one. Our death is inevitable.

On death, we must also consider the downward steps most of us will take on the way to our final breath, particularly as we are living an average of 50% longer than those born before 1900. What are those steps? Decline and disability. 80% of us will die in an institution like a nursing home or hospital. 20% will die at home. In the year 1900, these figures were reversed with 80% of people dying younger, at home, and 20% dying in institutions. There will be a period of your life, of undefined time, where you and I are likely to be under the care of others. In the West, there is a high chance we will spend some of our sunset years in an 'age ghetto' (residential aged care facilities), because those in our lives don't have the ability or time to care for us. Today, the average length of time someone lives in end-of-life aged care before dying is 22 months. As time passes, a percentage of us will experience cognitive decline and live with dementia. Over time, a good number of us won't be able to walk. Others will live months and years with disabilities and conditions that keep us wheelchair-bound or bed-ridden. Relative strangers in the form of care staff will wash us, feed us, protect us, medicate us, and keep us alive. These are all kinds of deaths. Death to our memory, death to our mobility, death to our privacy, death to our dignity, death to our pride. And all this will happen; it's just a matter of time.

One of my favourite authors, Dr. John Swinton, reminds us that time is not a force to be conquered but a friend to be met. In 'Becoming Friends of Time' (2018), Swinton speaks of a different way of dwelling in time – one that is not ruled by speed or productivity but by presence, relationship, and grace. To sit with the dying rather than rush past them, to honour the slow work of grief, to dwell in the present with those who have forgotten the past through cognitive decline - **this** is the invitation of "timefullness" is not about **doing** more but about **being** more **in** time. It is about walking at the pace of love rather than the demands of industry and progress.

So, we see that time and death, though deep friends, are not enemies of life. They are guides, asking us to walk more gently and be present to moments. Decentric elders have made friends with time and death. To befriend them both is to surrender to their mystery, to notice, to listen, to love, and in doing so, perhaps learn what it means to truly live.

*You have more*
*to offer*
*than an*
*un-grieved return*
*to your former,*
*younger life*

*The world*
*needs wisdom,*
*yours, now,*
*not winding back.*

*Do not return*
*to the ground*
*laying down*
*for the last time*
*as a stifled soul*
*stuck in an aged body.*

*Endure the dark night.*
*Heed the descending call.*
*Shed the coat of many colours.*
*Brighten the world*
*with your stained smile.*

*Make the mature choice*
*to mature well*
*as you tread lighter*
*across the earth*
*in your weathered*
*body-home*
*into the present day*
*as your present*
*and sober*
*eldering*
*self.*

*'What You Have to Offer'*
*David Tensen (2025)*

# Questions for reflection and discussion.

How might parenting and caregiving serve as "a decades-long apprenticeship in self-forgetting"? How does this perspective challenge contemporary views of parenting?

Where do you see evidence of death denial in your everyday life and cultural practices?

How might accepting the reality of death transform your approach to living and ageing?

What might it mean that "Death is one of the most real moments of your life" in practical terms?

What "deaths" might you experience before physical death (loss of mobility, privacy, independence)? How might accepting these "deaths" contribute to authentic eldering, as this book advocates?

How might "gerotranscendence" (described as "a natural shift from a materialistic and rational perspective towards a more cosmic and transcendent worldview") relate to your approach to death?

How might befriending time rather than fighting against it transform your experience of ageing?

# DECENTER CONSUMPTION

I have left this 'Decenter…' chapter until last because it may be the most challenging. And if you've come this far in the book, I can only suspect you are getting something from it, and are perhaps provoked towards action and change. The difficulty with writing about wealth and material assets for me is that unlike social, emotional, and spiritual capital, I have not accumulated much material wealth across my adult life. While writing this, I still rent my home. The cars in our carport are simple old 2001 and 2011 Toyotas. As mentioned previously, I went into voluntary bankruptcy in my 30s. Compared to my family and friends I went to school with, my superannuation and monetary wealth portfolio is fractional. Spending much of your life in service to others, through the church and charities, is rarely the road to 'financial independence'. Living on one income because of an invisible injury Natalie lived with for over a decade didn't help either. Add to this the damaging effects of the 'prosperity gospel' I was exposed to as a young Christian, and you have an Aussie guy in his 50s, significantly behind the wealthy middle-aged white guy wealth pack. I've had to push back against Western cultural ideologies of success and safety daily. I'm still working on it, but to a large extent, I have made peace with it all. The financial and vocational decisions I have made in life **are what they are**. They have been both necessary and soul-led. My material world isn't extravagant, but my inner life and connection to the Source of life is incredibly rich. And now, decades into life, and working among the aged, I can see how burdensome, destructive, and dizzying material wealth can be, later in life. I want to suggest to you that the practice of decentric eldering is not one focused on accumulation, but one mindful of distribution. It's not about growing deeper roots and wider branches, but about shedding leaves and seeds for those in our shade and care – whatever that looks like – preferably while we are still around to celebrate and guide the fruit it bears.

Around the world, societies have structured the transition from life's accumulative years to the distributive phase in different ways. In the West, retirement in later years typically centers on individual security and leisure. We're expected to gather sufficient personal wealth to fund decades of self-directed activities like travel and camping. Meanwhile, throughout East Asia, ageing follows a more relational pattern with elders remaining integrated in family structures, often living with adult children, and participating actively in raising grandchildren. Many Indigenous traditions position elders as cultural custodians rather than retirees. For example, many Aboriginal and Torres Strait Islander communities in Australia recognise Elders as knowledge-holders with responsibility for cultural continuity. And in Nordic countries, strong welfare states provide universal security for ageing citizens, creating psychological space for civic engagement without existential anxiety.

Each cultural approach has its benefits and drawbacks, so I'm not suggesting we all jump ship to adopt a culture outside our own. I hope by now you see that decentric eldering is a contextual practice. However, we can only decenter what we can see, and mammon is a god the colonial West has sacrificed to for centuries. Research in the field of cross-cultural gerontology (the study of ageing people) consistently shows differences in wellbeing outcomes across different cultural approaches.

Older persons in more collectivist culture, like those in Asia, often report different patterns of life satisfaction compared to those in individualistic societies. The Western model's emphasis on independence may inadvertently undermine psychological health by reducing natural support systems. In classic terms, you can gain the world, but it will cost you your soul and all that your soul was created to enjoy.

The call to decenter consumption isn't a judgement on any particular cultural approach, nor on any dollar value, but rather an invitation to conscious discernment. It asks us to examine whether our relationship to material resources reflects our deepest values or merely unconscious invisible conditioning. Do we not receive constant affirmation for maximising retirement accounts, purchasing retirement properties, and planning for decades of leisure? These actions aren't inherently problematic, but they often overshadow alternative possibilities for meaningful autumn and winter stages of life. The constant media bombardment of retirement as a time of luxurious travel, unending leisure, and material comfort rarely mentions the psychological emptiness many retirees experience after the initial honeymoon period ends.

Consider what happens in a typical Western retirement scenario. After decades of identity formation around productive work and raising families, many older adults find themselves adrift in an unfamiliar landscape where their primary focus becomes consumption and self-preservation. People go from careers and family roles where they managed, met, and served society, to a kind of self-service mode of being. The retired accountant, teacher, plumber or nurse go from changing lives to managing fluctuating retirement funds, medical appointments, sports events, and planning cruise and caravanning itineraries. These transitions aren't inherently wrong, but most often they represent a narrowing rather than an expansion of purpose. It's as if, in cultures like my own, the esteemed and default life looks like freedom and dreams without much money in our teens, to four decades of hard labour, so we can be teens again, but now with money, thinning hair, and backs that eventually go out more often than we do. Of course, this isn't true for everyone. Death, divorce, disability, and decay all diminish many of these cultural dreams – leaving many feeling like failures and 'less than'. Sadly, in Australia right now, women over 55 are among the fastest growing homeless demographic.

There is a tragedy to modern retirement ideology. Just when older people have the most to give, the cultural script suggests they should primarily take for themselves. This mismatch creates a developmental bottleneck where gifts that could flow into the community remain blocked. Decentric elders move naturally towards generativity and cultural contribution, where the focus shifts from personal achievement to creating lasting value for future generations.

Financial advisors routinely share stories of clients with millions in superannuation who live in constant fear of running out, unable to enjoy what they have or share it meaningfully with others. This isn't prudence; it's a pathology born of deep-seated insecurity and a culture that measures success in accumulated currency rather than altruistic contribution.

The shortsightedness among many of those who have accumulated material wealth in our day is troubling. Decentric elders understand that no one accumulates wealth or status through pure individual effort. All our achievements (and failures) emerge through complex systems of support: family networks, educational institutions, community infrastructure, economic systems, and cultural frameworks. The successful business builder benefited from public education, stable markets, favourable politics, employees' labour, community infrastructure, and countless other social goods. The healthcare professional relied on universities, research communities, colleagues, and patients willing to trust their expertise. The property developer utilised public roads, planning frameworks, tradespersons' skills, and financing systems that made their work possible. To be very blunt here: The myth of the self-made man (or woman) is among the dumbest and most dangerous modern ideologies. It carries a stench of pride, violence, and absolute self-centered ignorance.

Maturation involves recognising our utter interdependence, and therefore engages in conscious reciprocity. This might mean making financial contributions to institutions that provide opportunities, mentoring younger generations in your field, volunteering skills and expertise to community organisations, or supporting family members navigating their own life transitions. It could involve establishing scholarships, funding community initiatives, preserving natural spaces, or creating structural supports for vulnerable populations.

There is substantial evidence supporting the benefits of such giving and divestment of resources. Various studies examining volunteering behaviour among older adults show connections between regular contribution and reduced depressive symptoms, lower mortality rates, and higher life satisfaction. I'm told this holds true even when controlling for baseline health factors. Older persons who give the most of themselves often exhibit the greatest vitality and purpose.

On a broader scale, the developmental paradox appears clear: giving resources away like time, money, wisdom, and attention correlates with increased wellbeing. This isn't mystical or magical thinking, but the natural outcome of aligning with our inherently relational nature. Humans evolved in tight-knit communities where elders contributed wisdom and resources rather than withdrawing into isolated leisure. When we act in accordance with our relational design, we thrive. Just as trees in autumn release their leaves, giving back to the soil the nutrients they've gathered, human development should naturally move towards dispensing rather than accumulating. We see this pattern in healthy ecosystems everywhere: nothing hoards indefinitely. Surplus is released. Resources flow, cycle, and transform.

*Blessed*

*beyond measure*

*is the one found planted*

*in a field among generous friends.*

*Like great oaks, every act of kindness*

*sown to the soil strengthens the forest floor,*

*their nourishing*

*Roots*

*Grafting*

*As*

*One*

*To*

*weather every season's storm.*

'*Generous Friends*'

*David Tensen*

*The Saving I Need (2021)*

Hear me out, especially those prone to an all-or-nothing approach to life: this divestment and sowing into the soil is not about forced asceticism or denial of comfort, but about the deep satisfaction that comes with aligning with life's natural rhythms. Decentric Elders know that the process of intentional divestment - of possessions, roles, identities, and attachments that no longer serve, can create space for new growth, even as physical capacities diminish.

If divestment is not your default posture, and you tend to hoard out of greed, fear, or a sense of justice, the next steps for you may be approached as an experiment, to begin with. You see, acts of distribution and divestment help align your relationship to the healthy flow of life. Rivers that don't flow become stagnant. Compost that is not agitated rots and smells. For you, this might mean giving away valuable objects, sharing financial resources, volunteering time, or offering expertise; all without expectation of return. Pay attention to the heartfelt response in your innermost being. As the process deepens, practising different cultural forms of giving may prove valuable. While we shouldn't appropriate other cultural practices wholesale, we can learn from diverse approaches to sowing and divesting. Spend time with authentic elders from different cultural backgrounds, if you can. Read widely about ageing practices across societies. Visit communities where older people are playing integral roles. Who knows, you may even be empowered to decenter internalised Western ideologies of pseudo-eldering.

To clarify, the invitation of decentric eldering isn't a call to abandon material comfort or prudent planning, but to right-size these concerns within a more generous posture towards meaning and contribution. This practice asks us to consider whether our culture's obsession with individual security might actually be undermining the communal fabric that provides our deepest security. Echoed across history, research, religion, and within the laws of nature is this undeniable truth worth branding our hearts with: *the path of accumulation without divestment leads to a poverty of spirit and eventual extinction.*

As I write, Australia and other Western countries are facing a housing shortage. Housing affordability has become a leading topic in political discussions and remains a very complex and nuanced issue. Suffice to say that young adults, whom two decades ago would have left home by the time they were 20, are still living at home and simply have to stay at home longer in order to afford living. Intergenerational living is not a new concept, but as I touched on in the opening chapters, over the last century we have gone through such an economic and population boom that the dispersion and independence of families has been normalised. I believe multigenerational homes will be far more common in the West in the decades to come.

Of course, multigenerational living is not new to many cultures and families. When I speak to my Asian and Middle Eastern colleagues and friends about multigenerational living, they laugh and tell me how normal it is to live with your parents and grandparents in multigenerational homes. Today, however, it seems as though a man in his mid-twenties or thirties in Australia, the US, Canada, or the UK is publicly mocked and memed if he still lives at home with his parents – particularly 'in the basement'.

With the cost of living and the cost of housing four to five times what it was just a few decades ago, so many people will not be given the choice but to live in multigenerational homes. Not just because children can't afford it, but also because parents will also struggle to afford a mortgage, rent or otherwise, on their own. I think this is one of the reasons that decentering everything in our lives is going to be important because the question of 'Who are we to become?' isn't simply for those over 70. The question I'm asking myself as I approach 50 and have a 15, 17, and 21-year-old at home is, "Am I the sort of person that can live in a multigenerational home?" I can tell you now that the individualistic mindset that has permeated the West and driven us all into our individual castles and wealth that is not shared among generations is coming back to bite us. In fact, fractured families, disgruntled children, estranged parents, and epidemics of loneliness have been eating away at our society for quite some time.

Right now, I am asking myself other questions too:

Am I the kind of person that my children or my grandchildren could or would want to live with?

Will I be competition for my grandchildren when it comes to housing, jobs, and economic support?

Will I demand my own time, my own space, my own success?

Will I be willing to leave a career, money, promise, and accolades to care for my future generations?

Am I willing to give away any of 'my' fortunes before I die? Or will they need to be pried from disabled and dead hands?

Yes, in part, this is a callback to a collective society where things like the Hero's Journey are not individual journeys. Instead, they are collective adventures. They are tales of family dynasties. They are generations in harmony with what it means to be human. They are people who clearly understand that perceived threats to our lifestyle are vastly different from real threats upon our lives.

# Questions for reflection and discussion.

What might you learn from diverse cultural approaches to ageing - from Western individualism to Asian familial integration to Indigenous cultural custodianship?

How have you witnessed the mismatch where "just when older people have got the most to give, the cultural script suggests they should primarily take for themselves"?

How might you challenge the "myth of the self-made individual" in your own thinking?

What implications does this chapter have for your approach to wealth and resources, if any?

What evidence have you seen that "giving resources away like time, money, wisdom, and attention correlates with gaining well-being"?

What might a practice "not of accumulation, but of distribution" look like in practical terms in your life or community?

How does the rise of multigenerational homes challenge your assumptions about independence in later life?

If you asked yourself: "Am I the kind of person that my children or my grandchildren could or would want to live with?", how might you answer?

# WHERE TO FROM HERE?

Given the statistics on the average number of pages a person reads in a book, if you have come this far, thank you so much. I certainly hope that this little manifesto has provoked your thinking in some way, even if your thinking might be, 'David's gone mad, and lost the plot.'

But seriously, in this closing chapter, I want to recap and highlight some of the previous points and share my heart on the way forward. We opened with an overview of the place we find ourselves today, in a society full of wonderful older persons, lacking the kind of psycho-social-spiritually mature elders we need and seek. I also suggested that these kinds of elders are not necessarily constrained by age, nor do cultural and institutional titles define them. Instead, they are soulmakers who emerge and mature over decades.

I acknowledge that, perhaps for some, kicking off with decentering God is the hardest of all decentered movements – more challenging than being heard, more difficult that acquiring knowledge, more significant than death, and more pressing than accumulation. But perhaps you are one of the few who grasped that true union cannot exist while we center our construct of God in our life, or center ourselves in God's life as more exceptional and special than others (including our enemies). If you see no disharmony or dichotomy between these two, I respect that. Personally, however, I believe that we can only move forward with a loving gaze and capacity to hold all things if we **become like God** (theosis) by accepting the mystical and unconditional gift of union with Christ who exists and enjoys the self-emptying loving communion of the Trinity.

Believe me when I say that if you are actively pursuing God through any construct or way, the act of decentering God for the sake of union is one worth exploring, even on a daily basis. Perhaps here you might ask yourself, does the concept or construct of God that I have contain any unnecessary and unhelpful notions of alienation and separation? Or you might simply ask yourself, *how am I in union with God?* Perhaps you might even ask yourself if there is space and room for God to appear in a way that would hinder you from loving your neighbour as yourself?

I would argue that decentering being heard and making way for others through companioning is non-negotiable in the practice of decentric eldering. We must be willing to relinquish the role of the hero in our own journey so that we do not fall prey to center-stage syndrome, particularly in the second half of life.

If you are reading this and you are in the first half of life, in the spring and summer seasons, it is important that you understand and walk out the Hero's Journey. As Richard Rohr and others point out, we should avoid demonising the formation of our identity in the first half of life, and we should also avoid demonising our ego. It is essential that we come to know our strengths and weaknesses, and that we come to know what we are capable of. We should build resilience, build character, build determination, live with goals and dreams, and more. The first half of life is for this.

If you were fortunate enough to either grow up in a functional home or move with great success from dysfunctional to functioning somewhere earlier in life, perhaps in your twenties and thirties, then you'll know how important a sense of order and certainty is to who we are. Living with self-doubt, low self-esteem, self-hatred, poor boundaries, and subsequent mental health challenges that can make the Hero's Journey a challenging or distressing one. Regardless, there comes a time when we all must decenter ourselves. Decenter unnecessary stories. Decenter the need to remain a hero. Decenter the need to become and remain an expert. Decenter the importance of being heard. Decenter becoming the sage-on-the-stage and instead say 'yes' to the invitation to being the guide-on-the-side. To be the companion who is not there to fix, is not there to take over or dominate, to coerce or control, but instead to be a humble witness and friend for others along a portion of another's life, as they walk their own journey.

Acquiring knowledge to make room for true wisdom often comes by grace and the outworking of the cliché, *the older I get, the less I know.* Wisdom, as you will have read, differs from knowledge and the decentric elder is called to be a wisdom-holder and not a knowledge-dispenser. In our digital age, we certainly do not need the simple repetition of facts or cognitive parroting. The world needs a blend of experience, capacity and knowledge. We need embodied decentered others – those who are not simply information carriers but souls who are peace-filled, self-forgetting, self-emptying and source-full.

Is it any wonder that the work of Jesus Christ includes the overcoming of death? He lived in a time and society where death was on display, including the sacrificial death of animals at temples, or the youthful death and treatment of bodies in His day. Decentric elders have broken free from the denial of death. They understand it is coming, and have accepted that they should not fight time but befriend it, recognising that every day, right up to their last, is truly a gift.

Finally, decentering accumulation is perhaps one of the most pervasive and difficult messages for some in the West. But as you've just read in the last chapter, I would argue that decentric elders understand the time and season they're in, and are willing to adjust lifestyle expectations, give of themselves, and divest that which they have in abundance, including material wealth.

Please understand, this book is by no means designed to be the final word on the topic of elderhood, but a voice amongst voices. However, I do feel there is a sense of urgency for discussions like this to be had. Considerations on how we might continue to **grow up** throughout our lifespan into our older years are important. But I cannot overstate the importance of remembering that, historically, we have not been here before.

We have not been in this economy before; we have not been in this world of information before; we have certainly not lived en masse this long before. I am not keen on adding to the constant onslaught of real or imagined crisis that the mass media, politicians, and economists use to garner attention. Still, I believe there will be a heavy price to pay if people like myself, in mid-life, expect to live out our days with the same kind of socially supported and funded lifestyle our parents and grandparents' generation did. We owe it to those before us to evolve into the kind of people that leave a legacy that challenges over-consumption, challenges harmful notions of success and progress, and makes an effort to repair our collective connection to the actual planet that we live in.

Author Bill Plotkin reminds us of how ridiculous the simple idea of *getting back to nature is,* given that **we are all part of nature**. I need not remind us of how a simple germ, disease, or biological force can transform our lives. COVID-19 and our relationship to it, with all its losses and trauma, are a recent demonstration of that.

We cannot continue on as a species who sees ourselves separate from nature and the environment.

I know I keep repeating this point, but it should be said that being heard, knowledge, death, and material gain are all important, however; they cannot remain at the center of our lives, they must all be decentered along with everything else.

We must now reimagine what eldering will look like in the coming decades, in our time, as the population grows, as our environment and ecology groan, as our financial systems, mental health, and collective happiness decline. We have been presented with an opportunity to begin to reimagine what it might look like to live longer and in a healthier way than our predecessors, with immense generosity and fatness of soul. With an expanded capacity for wisdom, life, listening and divestment, I believe we can embrace the invitation to inhabit the (chronological) age that we each are and thoughtfully inhabit the period of history that we collectively live in.

This **is** the call to decentric eldering: **it is a call to true and honest inhabiting of our own age and the age that we live in.** And I truly believe the call can and should begin early in life. The eldering journey must transcend barriers of late-life chronological age proposed by gerontologists and be something our young people are on a journey towards, not unlike the generous discussions that prepare people for parenting today.

War, capitalism, technology, and a whole variety of reasons have brought us to this point in time where the kind of decentric elders I have described throughout the book are scarce, but it does not mean that we should keep walking down the same well-worn elderless path. We are now in a period of time where, as I wrote earlier, we must learn to elder without (many) elders.

We must break free from the self-centered, self-absorbed center-stage illusions others have sold us, which separate us from God. I'm very wary of considering myself any kind of ground-breaker or pioneer in this space, because so much of this book is borrowed and synthesised. I am simply continuing a conversation that has been had, and is being had, across different fields of study and thought.

The world needs decentric elders to emerge quietly on its fringes, not making a big deal about it all, but simply going about doing the work of divesting, loving, and creating belonging in the space and the time God has called them to inhabit. Over time, if we can do this, the fertile soil of wisdom traditions created will make way for a more generous and sustainable future.

Again, I would love to hear from you via david@davidtensen.com. I believe that we need to keep this conversation going. The QR code and URL will connect you to resources that will help you on your decentric eldering journey, including references, further readings, and ways to connect with others.


Much love.
David Tensen

www.davidtensen.com/decenter

References, Readings, Resources and More

# Closing questions for reflection and discussion.

Looking at the five areas you might need to decenter (God, being heard, knowledge, death, consumption), which do you find most challenging to decenter in your own life?

What would it mean for you to more fully inhabit both your current age and this historical moment? How might this dual inhabiting transform your experience?

How might the practice of decentric eldering begin earlier in life? What would this look like for younger generations?

Why might quietness and fringe positioning rather than centre-stage leadership be important in eldering?

What resources might support your learning to elder in the absence of strong elder models?

How has your understanding of elderhood shifted through your exploration of these ideas?

What concrete steps could you take to move towards decentric eldering in your own life?

# Other books by David Tensen

The Wrestle (2020)

So I Wrote You a Poem (2021)

The Saving I Need (2021)

Winters Never Last (2022)

The Kid Without a Costume (2024)

Decenter Everything (2025)

Find them at www.davidtensen.com
and online book retailers.

Enquiries: david@davidtensen.com

Printed in Dunstable, United Kingdom